Overcoming Common Problems Series

Coping with Macular Degeneration
Dr Patricia Gilbert

Coping with the Menopause
Janet Horwood

Coping with a Mid-life Crisis
Derek Milne

Coping with Polycystic Ovary Syndrome
Christine Craggs-Hinton

Coping with Postnatal Depression
Sandra L. Wheatley

Coping with SAD
Fiona Marshall and Peter Cheevers

Coping with Snoring and Sleep Apnoea
Jill Eckersley

Coping with a Stressed Nervous System
Dr Kenneth Hambly and Alice Muir

Coping with Strokes
Dr Tom Smith

Coping with Suicide
Maggie Helen

Coping with Thyroid Problems
Dr Joan Gomez

Curing Arthritis – The Drug-Free Way
Margaret Hills

Curing Arthritis Diet Book
Margaret Hills

Curing Arthritis Exercise Book
Margaret Hills and Janet Horwood

Depression
Dr Paul Hauck

Depression at Work
Vicky Maud

Depressive Illness
Dr Tim Cantopher

Eating Disorders and Body Image
Christine Craggs-Hinton

Eating for a Healthy Heart
Robert Povey, Jacqui Morrell and Rachel Povey

Effortless Exercise
Dr Caroline Shreeve

Fertility
Julie Reid

The Fibromyalgia Healing Diet
Christine Craggs-Hinton

Free Your Life from Fear
Jenny Hare

Getting a Good Night's Sleep
Fiona Johnston

Heal the Hurt: How to Forgive and Move On
Dr Ann Macaskill

Heart Attacks – Prevent and Survive
Dr Tom Smith

Help Your Child Get Fit Not Fat
Jan Hurst and Sue Hubberstey

Helping Children Cope with Anxiety
Jill Eckersley

Helping Children Cope with Change and Loss
Rosemary Wells

Helping Children Get the Most from School
Sarah Lawson

How to Be Your Own Best Friend
Dr Paul Hauck

How to Beat Pain
Christine Craggs-Hinton

How to Cope with Bulimia
Dr Joan Gomez

How to Cope with Difficult People
Alan Houel and Christian Godefroy

How to Improve Your Confidence
Dr Kenneth Hambly

How to Keep Your Cholesterol in Check
Dr Robert Povey

How to Stick to a Diet
Deborah Steinberg and Dr Windy Dryden

How to Stop Worrying
Dr Frank Tallis

Hysterectomy
Suzie Hayman

The Irritable Bowel Diet Book
Rosemary Nicol

Is HRT Right for You?
Dr Anne MacGregor

Letting Go of Anxiety and Depression
Dr Windy Dryden

Lifting Depression the Balanced Way
Dr Lindsay Corrie

Living with Alzheimer's Disease
Dr Tom Smith

Living with Asperger Syndrome
Dr Joan Gomez

Living with Asthma
Dr Robert Youngson

Living with Autism
Fiona Marshall

Overcoming Common Problems Series

Living with Crohn's Disease
Dr Joan Gomez

Living with Diabetes
Dr Joan Gomez

Living with Fibromyalgia
Christine Craggs-Hinton

Living with Food Intolerance
Alex Gazzola

Living with Grief
Dr Tony Lake

Living with Heart Disease
Victor Marks, Dr Monica Lewis and
Dr Gerald Lewis

Living with High Blood Pressure
Dr Tom Smith

Living with Hughes Syndrome
Triona Holden

Living with Loss and Grief
Julia Tugendhat

Living with Lupus
Philippa Pigache

Living with Nut Allergies
Karen Evennett

Living with Osteoarthritis
Dr Patricia Gilbert

Living with Osteoporosis
Dr Joan Gomez

Living with Rheumatoid Arthritis
Philippa Pigache

Living with Sjögren's Syndrome
Sue Dyson

Losing a Baby
Sarah Ewing

Losing a Child
Linda Hurcombe

**Make Up or Break Up: Making the Most of
Your Marriage**
Mary Williams

Making Friends with Your Stepchildren
Rosemary Wells

Making Relationships Work
Alison Waines

Overcoming Anger
Dr Windy Dryden

Overcoming Anxiety
Dr Windy Dryden

Overcoming Back Pain
Dr Tom Smith

Overcoming Depression
Dr Windy Dryden and Sarah Opie

Overcoming Impotence
Mary Williams

Overcoming Jealousy
Dr Windy Dryden

**Overcoming Loneliness and Making
Friends**
Márianna Csóti

Overcoming Procrastination
Dr Windy Dryden

Overcoming Shame
Dr Windy Dryden

The PMS Diet Book
Karen Evennett

Rheumatoid Arthritis
Mary-Claire Mason and Dr Elaine Smith

The Self-Esteem Journal
Alison Waines

Shift Your Thinking, Change Your Life
Mo Shapiro

Stress at Work
Mary Hartley

Ten Steps to Positive Living
Dr Windy Dryden

Think Your Way to Happiness
Dr Windy Dryden and Jack Gordon

The Traveller's Good Health Guide
Ted Lankester

**Understanding Obsessions and
Compulsions**
Dr Frank Tallis

When Someone You Love Has Depression
Barbara Baker

Your Man's Health
Fiona Marshall

Overcoming Common Problems

Living with Lupus

Philippa Pigache

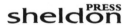

First published in Great Britain in 2005

Sheldon Press
36 Causton Street
London SW1P 4ST

Copyright © Philippa Pigache 2005

The author and publisher have made every effort to ensure that the external website
and email addresses included in this book are correct and up to date at the time of
going to press. The author and publisher are not responsible for the content, quality
or continuing accessibility of the sites.

British Library Cataloguing-in-Publication Data

A catalogue record for this book is available from the British Library

ISBN 0–85969–952–8

1 3 5 7 9 10 8 6 4 2

Typeset by Deltatype Limited, Birkenhead, Merseyside
Printed in Great Britain by
Ashford Colour Press

To my colleague and friend Tom Smith,
who held my hand on the wolf-hunt

Contents

Introduction – the wolf and the butterfly

What is Lupus? Ask the medical experts and they will tell you it is an *autoimmune disease*. Its full name is *systemic lupus erythematosus*, or SLE, though we will be referring to it as 'lupus' for short. The 'systemic' indicates that it affects many organs – the whole system. The 'erythematosus' – from the Greek word for red – describes a certain kind of rash and refers to the part of the body most noticeably affected in lupus: the skin. Until the nineteenth century, lupus was thought of only as a skin disease. In fact the name was almost certainly applied to other diseases affecting the skin on the face, not to what we know as lupus today.

'Lupus' is the Latin for wolf and the name was coined seven centuries ago by the medieval physicians Rogerius and Paracelsus to describe facial lesions that 'ate' into the skin, and looked like a wolf bite. These days, doctors think it more likely that such lesions were caused by a form of tuberculosis, rather than what we now call lupus.

In the past it was also sometimes called lupus vulgaris, or common lupus. This was to distinguish it from a slightly different kind of rash – raised circular discs – which was called discoid lupus for obvious reasons, and which is now considered to be a different version of the same disease – systemic lupus erythematosus.

So forget about the wolf. Think instead of the butterfly. This delightful creature is used accurately to describe a characteristic rash that appears on the faces of many people with lupus, spreading from the bridge of the nose to fan out across the cheeks (in colouration anything from rose pink to angry red) – erythematosus.

The fact that the illness affected other organs was not appreciated until the end of the nineteenth century. At this time it was discovered that lupus involved inflammation of the joints – *arthritis* – fatigue, and a number of other physical symptoms including potentially fatal kidney damage.

Once the link between the skin rash and fatal kidney disease had been established, lupus got a very bad press. Medical textbooks printed in the first half of the twentieth century spoke of it with gloom and despondency. Women – 90 per cent of sufferers are women of childbearing age – were warned against getting pregnant or going out in the sun and given a generally depressing prognosis. Sadly there are still a few medical persons who cleave to this opinion.

If you or someone you love has lupus, I am pleased to inform you that this is total, old-fashioned rubbish. Before there were refined laboratory tests to identify the condition, the only cases that were recognized were those of people who had had the disease severely and had remained untreated for many years. Now that it is usually diagnosed and treated, it emerges that many more people suffer, but quite mildly. In fact the current belief is that there are thousands of 'sleeping' lupus sufferers who go peacefully to their graves for some quite unrelated cause, unaware that they have ever had it.

Those whose condition is diagnosed cannot yet be offered a cure, but increased understanding of what goes on in the disease, combined with modern treatment, takes the bite out of lupus. The wolf may not be dying out, but it is certainly a much less threatening creature than thought to be in the past.

Nevertheless lupus is still a mysterious illness. Like its namesake, it lurks in the shadows of the forest and comes out at night to leave unexplained damage and devastation. And, like the animal in the fable wearing sheep's clothing, it is difficult to recognize and often gets mistaken for something else. We hope this book will explain some of the mysteries surrounding lupus.

Hints for the reader

You can read this book from beginning to end, or simply dip in and out, picking out what interests or concerns you. Only the first two chapters, which explain the key features of lupus, are essential to understanding the rest of the book. The chapters (4 and 5) on diagnosis are important if you think you, or someone close to you, may be a sufferer, and the chapters (6, 7 and 8) on treatment and management are important for someone already confirmed with lupus. I have tried to use cross-headings and titles that will help you find what you are in search of (or see the index), or to skip what you don't need to read.

Difficult words are explained in the text and those printed in *italic type* when first they appear (though not throughout the text) are also listed in the glossary at the end of the book. Some interesting information on the general story of lupus is picked out in separate boxes.

1
Recognizing lupus – the wolf's spoor

First thing in the morning you peer into the mirror and there is a bright, red rash. From the bridge of your nose it spreads to cover both cheeks in the classic shape of a butterfly. If you had spent all yesterday unprotected in bright sunlight you might wonder if you had caught the sun, but most probably you would think, 'Heavens! I've caught something. Was it something I ate?'

That's the thing about skin. It's the largest organ of the body and, being on the outside, is extremely noticeable. As teenagers we subjected every pimple, lump or blemish to minute examination and they filled us with anxiety. As adults we learn to take the odd spot, bruise or wrinkle in our stride, but a rash is something different. Perhaps it is our recollection of childhood ailments like measles or chickenpox, familiar even in these days of immunization; perhaps it is the association between rash and eating or touching something dangerous, or even a dim folk memory of historic but fatal epidemics like smallpox or the plague. Either way we know, almost instinctively, that a rash is a sign of something wrong. If it's on your face you can't ignore it. If it sticks around for some days, you will almost certainly take it to the doctor.

This is why the oldest recognized symptom of lupus is a rash. Other symptoms may be explained away, ignored or not recognized as being part of an illness, but a rash on the face merits some sort of attention.

The multiple personality of lupus

But the butterfly has many faces. Suppose that instead of a rash you wake in the morning with inexplicable fever, headache or fatigue. Suppose every joint and muscle in your body seems to ache. Suppose your eyes are dry and scratchy or your hair comes out in chunks on your comb. Suppose your ankles get puffy, or that you become so depressed you feel life is hardly worth living. Would you conclude that you had something serious? Would you think it worth bothering the doctor? Or would you decide that you were a bit run down or starting a cold, and take a few days off in the hope that it might all blow over?

1

This is why the multiple manifestations of lupus took so long to become recognized. Lupus is systemic – that is, it affects many organs throughout the body; and lupus is *chronic*: it comes and goes. Left untreated it may afflict you for a period of days or weeks but then may inexplicably clear up and leave you in peace for months or even years. To begin with there is no permanent damage; the temperature goes down, your skin clears, the aches and pains go away and the hair grows again. There may be clues that all is not well – the rash may flare if you are out in the sun; other symptoms recur if you eat certain foods or go through a period of stress. You begin to notice that your body has started reacting to things that didn't bother it before. But it is perfectly possible to live with the wolf for years without knowing it.

By describing it as chronic and systemic we explain when and where lupus occurs. By classifying it as an autoimmune disease we indicate which body system underlies what goes wrong in lupus. We will explore this in more detail in Chapter 3. Put simply, in lupus part of the body's defence system (*antibodies*) normally produced to ward off foreign invaders like bacteria or viruses, starts misbehaving, and attacks the body's own tissues.

There are other diseases in which the body's defence system runs amok; most of them have only recently begun to be understood – and even then imperfectly. The best known is type 1 diabetes where part of the immune system destroys the cells that manufacture insulin, a hormone the body needs to break down the sugars in food to supply energy. Autoimmune cells are also involved in some cancers like *leukaemia* but, more significantly for people with lupus, they are implicated in *rheumatoid arthritis* – a disease closely related to lupus and sometimes mistaken for it.

Naming lupus families and relations

Once you know which family lupus comes from, and who some of its close relations are, it becomes easier to understand why it is so easily mistaken for other similar diseases. Lupus forms part of a big family called *connective tissue diseases*: CTD for short. Connective tissue is present all over the body, which is why the symptoms of lupus are so diffuse. It includes skin, and also the lining or sheath of joints, tendons, ligaments, blood vessels, nerves and major organs

2

like the heart and lungs. Arthritis, the name for conditions that affect joints (*arthros* is Greek for joint), is the best-known member of the family. There are over one hundred forms of arthritis alone, so they might better be known in the plural as arthrit*es*. Other CTDs are systemic *sclerosis* (from the Greek word for hardening), which affects skin and connective tissue all over the body, *polymyositis* and *dermatomyositis* (these are conditions involving the inflammation of various muscles – Greek: *myo*, and skin: *derma)* or PM-DM, plus a host of other rare individual disorders or syndromes which have been identified but are too confusing to list here. (We look at them in more detail in Chapter 9.) There are CTDs that defy any of the established labels which the doctors call 'mixed connective tissue disease' or MCTD.

Medical specialists who treat lupus

Because lupus affects so many different parts of the body, a sufferer can come into contact with a vast array of medical specialists. Immunologists specialize in the immune system. Dermatologists treat skin diseases. *Rheumatologists* specialize in diseases that cause inflammation: lupus is a form of arthritis caused by inflammation. An *ophthalmologist* – a specialist in conditions of the eye – may be consulted if the eyes are affected, or a *nephrologist* – a kidney specialist – because, in its worst manifestations, lupus can damage the kidneys and if the disease affects the membranes that enclose the heart or lungs, a cardiologist may be consulted. If a lupus sufferer becomes pregnant she may develop a blood disorder and need to consult a *haematologist* (*haem* or *aem* in a medical word is from the Greek for blood). Many lucky lupus sufferers never get referred to specialists, but remain in the care of their family doctor, but even these will need the services of a hospital laboratory pathologist who specializes in analysing the sophisticated tests that tell you what's wrong and how treatment is progressing. (You can look up these and other medical terms in the glossary at the end of the book.)

It's all very confusing. And the reason is that connective tissue is ubiquitous – found all over the body – leading not only to a vast range of individual symptoms that may characterize each disease, but to a wide overlap of symptoms between CTDs. North American and European medical institutions have gone some way to inscribing diagnostic criteria in stone, but at the final count the naming of diseases is an imperfect science. In many cases uncertainty prevails, frustrating for both patient and doctor.

It may seem pointless, frivolous even to waste time and effort over precise medical labelling: what doctors refer to as establishing a *differential diagnosis*. But it has a vital role when it comes to deciding what treatment is likely to work and what outcome to expect.

Presenting symptoms: the patient's view

There are two ways of considering symptoms: the patient's view and the doctor's. They obviously overlap, but their significance is viewed differently. The patient has the intimate, day-to-day experience of living in his or her body: sometimes it feels better than others; there are all sorts of minor aches and pains, bumps or blemishes that come and go, signifying nothing. How they are rated depends more on whether the sufferer is a bit of a hypochondriac or frightfully British and stiff-upper-lip about things, no matter how severe or inconvenient they are.

Doctors know this and do their best to make allowances for it. They get to know that Mrs Wickins thinks she has developed an allergy every time she has a touch of indigestion whereas they don't see poor old Major Thomas until he has taken to his bed with pneumonia. But the patient's variable response to illness is a particular problem for doctors when the disease in question slips in and out of the forest every now and then leaving almost no trail, like lupus.

Janet's story
Janet discovered she had lupus when she became pregnant in her late twenties in 1978. 'You name a complication of pregnancy; I had it,' she says; 'blood clots, raised blood pressure, *oedema* (puffiness caused by fluid retention) up to my knees. And then a blood clot started blocking my heart. My obstetrician said I was lucky to have survived the pregnancy and that I should not risk another one.' Fortunately he also asked Janet several probing questions and discovered that as a teenager she had suffered from

4

a short attack of painfully swollen hands which her GP had put down to rheumatoid arthritis. She also told him that she had developed curious lumps in her legs when she had taken the birth control pill. The obstetrician said she might have 'collagen disease' and recommended that she see a rheumatologist. Janet was fortunate that by this time laboratory tests had been developed that provided a more conclusive diagnosis than the one offered by the shifting kaleidoscope of symptoms found with CTDs. Systemic lupus was diagnosed and by the time Janet was ready to undertake another pregnancy her doctors made sure she received treatment that prevented all the previous complications.

Let us look at lupus symptoms as the patient experiences them:

Malaise

Malaise is a French word for feeling generally unwell and uncomfortable. It has that 'can't put your finger on it' character that makes it likely to be ignored as a significant symptom of real illness. It may be accompanied by a slightly raised temperature or a headache. This malaise, with or without fever, is the commonest feature of lupus and probably, when the patient comes to look back, the first they experienced, though they didn't identify it at the time. It is probably caused by the disseminated (widespread or systemic) nature of lupus. Connective tissues all over the body may be inflamed, some in the joints, others in the brain, which can lead to headaches or depression. They may also be *anaemic*; meaning that the supply of important oxygen and glucose-carrying red blood cells in their blood is depleted. If a person does go to the doctor with these symptoms the cause is easily missed, or mislabelled as 'post-viral', *myalgic encephalitis (ME)* – or glandular fever.

Skin rash

In fact only about a fifth of those with lupus experience the classic butterfly rash as their first symptom. Ultimately about half have it. Nevertheless, the skin is one of the organs most commonly involved in the illness. The rash doesn't hurt or itch, though it may burn slightly if exposed to sunlight. In fact the lupus rash is a bit of a werewolf and takes several forms and appears in diverse places. It is sometimes faint and rosy and, because it often follows exposure to ultraviolet light, can occasionally be mistaken for sunburn. Other

5

times it takes the form of disc-shaped, scaly red patches which can appear anywhere on the body and which can leave scars when they clear up. They can occur in the scalp, causing hair loss which may be permanent. (Hair loss – which strictly speaking is another skin symptom – may occur in the absence of a rash. On those occasions it invariably regrows.) These raised plaques are the discoid lesions that occur in about 15 per cent of lupus sufferers, the vast majority of whom have none of the other lupus symptoms. For this reason it was, in the past, often classified as a separate illness – discoid lupus erythematosus. Because their symptoms are so mild it is likely that patients with discoid lesions slip between the population statistics of lupus, and in many parts of the world they may not even be seen by a doctor.

Sometimes the rash takes the form of small blisters *(vesicles)*. These may be on the face on the V-neck area, elbows, palms, tips of the fingers or the soles of the feet. In this last position it can easily be missed unless there are accompanying symptoms. The fluid-filled vesicles are caused by small blood vessels becoming inflamed and can appear on the finger tips or the elbows. Blisters can also crop up on the mouth taking the form of painless ulcers and occasionally in the vagina. About one in eight lupus patients have these at some time or other.

Faced with some of these varieties of rash a GP is on much firmer ground than with malaise. Lupus will definitely be among his or her likely suspects.

Before we leave skin manifestations of lupus it is worth mentioning a very common symptom: about a third of lupus patients are *photosensitive* – that is, they react in an extreme way to ultraviolet light with inflammation, burning and blistering. Some also react to fluorescent lights. This symptom has the advantage of being closely associated with lupus but with few other CTDs.

Arthritis

As we have heard in Janet's case (see page 4), lupus is easily mistaken for rheumatoid arthritis. As in this illness the joints most commonly affected are those of the hands, arms feet and legs. They are the first-noted symptom in about three-quarters of cases of lupus and most – in excess of 90 per cent – of diagnosed cases experience it at some time. The commonest pattern is for stiffness, tenderness and swelling of the fingers and wrists on waking. Unlike the joint pain in rheumatoid arthritis which in many cases is unremitting unless treated, lupus arthritis usually comes and goes and varies in intensity.

Shan's story

Shan worked in a busy insurance office and spent most of her time at the computer keyboard. She was 33 when she first noticed signs of arthritis – stiffness, swelling and pain – in her hands. 'Bit early for *osteoarthritis*', she said to herself. (Osteoarthritis is not caused by inflammation but mostly by normal wear and tear and doesn't usually show up until someone is in their fifties.) She also wondered about repetitive strain injury or carpal tunnel syndrome – two conditions that often bother people who type a lot. She took paracetamol and tried to ignore it. But then over a bank holiday she and her husband went walking in the Lake District. 'On the first day we must have covered 10 or 15 miles in a round trip. Something we could easily take in our stride, but the following morning I just couldn't get out of bed', she said. 'The weekend was ruined. The pain continued into the week. I couldn't go into work and ended up lying in bed with packs of frozen peas on my knees and ankles, unable to get up or go to sleep.' Shan's husband called the GP. The GP thought it was probably rheumatoid arthritis but when she took a history Shan remembered the mouth ulcers she had had a few years back. The GP sent off samples of Shan's blood to the laboratory and the results confirmed that it was lupus.

Heart and lung problems

The heart and lungs are both surrounded by membranes made of connective tissue. The heart membrane is called the *pericardium* and inflammation of the pericardium is called *pericarditis.* The equivalent membranes enclosing the lungs are called the *pleura* and inflammation of the pleura is *pleurisy.* When these membranes become inflamed the patient experiences pain, especially in breathing. These symptoms are unlikely to be the first experienced by anyone with lupus, but if they start out with fever and malaise, put it down to flu or a bad cold, things may escalate to bronchitis, pneumonia and then pleurisy. If things get to this stage the person will almost certainly be admitted to hospital and lots of tests will be done to identify the problem, resulting ultimately in an accurate diagnosis even if a number of others are considered first. As one patient put it: 'There isn't a single test that says unequivocally, "Yes, you have lupus." You sort of back into it after visiting several other possibilities.' Studies show that between 33 and 45 per cent of lupus sufferers have pleurisy at some time or other, and about 25 per cent may develop pericarditis.

Kidney problems

Half of those who have lupus develop some degree of kidney involvement at some stage. These symptoms, although unlikely to be among the first encountered by someone with lupus, can have a potentially fatal outcome. Prior to the 1940s, before modern understanding and modern drugs, it was kidney failure that gave lupus such a bad name. The person becomes aware of kidney problems in the form of puffy ankles, possibly puffy fingers and knees. When the kidneys are unable to filter waste products from the body adequately, fluid builds up, driven by gravity, from the ankles up. When fluid remains pooled in the tissues it causes swelling and discomfort called oedema. It is easy to identify because if you press a finger into the swelling the imprint does not fade for some minutes. Oedema is a signal that the kidneys are not coping. It is quite common in the latter stages of pregnancy even for women without lupus. It is confirmed by a simple urine test which detects the presence of protein fragments normally filtered out of the urine by healthy kidneys.

Blood problems

We have already mentioned that the malaise associated with lupus can partly be attributed to a shortage of red-blood cells – anaemia. Other blood cells may also be affected: white cells which fight off disease; or platelets, one of the mechanisms that cause blood to clot, may be in reduced supply. People are likely to feel tired (shortage of red cells), keep going down with minor ailments (shortage of white cells), or bruise easily (shortage of platelets) and heal slowly. Taken on their own, these symptoms may not convince someone they need to see their doctor. These only become significant when part of a larger picture. A laboratory test called a complete blood count (CBC) is needed to reveal that significance. One or other of these blood problems affects nearly all lupus patients at some time, though they are not necessarily the first symptoms the patient notices.

8

Up to here, some or all of these symptoms (some of which people may ignore or put down to the normal ups and downs of life) are the same as those the doctor needs to make a diagnosis of systemic lupus erythematosus.

Unlike a patient, limited to his or her own, subjective observations, doctors have more sophisticated ways of confirming or excluding various diseases. We will look at these laboratory tests when we return to diagnosis in Chapter 3.

Please note: all the symptoms of lupus listed here, with the possible exception of hair loss following discoid lesions, clear up with treatment leaving no damage.

Neither lupus, nor any other form of arthritis, is contagious, and having one kind does not predispose you to develop another.

2
Who develops lupus, where and why – the prey of the wolf

Damned lies or statistics

Estimates of noncontagious, nonreportable disease prevalence rely on some sort of official records such as hospital discharge logs, emergency-room visits, and reasons noted for school absences. It is thus possible to estimate number of heart attacks, broken legs and children suffering from severe asthma, for example, with reasonable accuracy.

Sheldon Paul Blau MD (see details of his book in 'Further reading')

These days we like numbers attached to illnesses. The science of who gets what, where and when is called *epidemiology*. It is not a very exact science. So where do we get these numbers from? If a disease is notifiable – in many countries doctors treating cases of serious or infectious diseases like tuberculosis must notify the authorities because there are public health consequences – accurate statistics on the incidence (number of new cases) of a disease can be assembled. Likewise, if a disease is fatal or puts you in hospital it then gets recorded as a cause of death or hospitalization and there may be a record of who succumbs to it – mortality and morbidity data (illness figures). However, lupus is not notifiable and only rarely is it fatal, so we learn little about it from these records. The reason it was rated potentially fatal in the past was that only serious and fatal cases of the disease were recorded. The large number of people who had lupus but didn't die of it, or even see a doctor about it, was unknown – like the body of a vast iceberg with only the fatal cases visible above the waterline.

Most experts believe that there are still many invisible, uncounted cases of lupus, particularly in underdeveloped countries with few doctors and more serious diseases to worry about, and estimates of the number of cases or the percentage of the population who develop lupus are constantly being revised upwards. The statistics that have been gathered relate mostly to developed countries with good health services and a network of medical laboratories and research institutes dedicated to the study of diseases and their treatment. In these countries scientists are funded to do population studies to ascertain who suffers from diseases, and statistics for the rest of the world are often extrapolations (scaled-up estimates) based on available studies. However, where lupus is concerned not all populations or geographic localities have the same experience.

Prevalence and incidence

In ordinary English we use these two words almost interchangeably. In statistics they measure two slightly different things. *Prevalence* usually refers to the estimated population of people suffering from a disease at any given time. *Incidence* refers to the number of new cases diagnosed each year. A short-lived disease like flu has a high annual incidence but low prevalence – people get it one after another but then get better. A lifelong disease like diabetes has a low annual incidence but high prevalence: only a few people develop it each year, but once they have it they have it for good. As lupus is chronic, new cases (incidence) may not add up perfectly into prevalence statistics.

Lupus occurs unevenly

In the total world population it has been calculated that something between forty and fifty people out of every thousand will have lupus at some time in their lives. These estimates have nearly tripled in the last forty years. This is probably not because the disease is actually on the increase, but because sophisticated immunological tests introduced in recent years, combined with improved diagnostic criteria, have led to mild cases of disease being recorded, so the estimates have been increased to allow for these cases.

In North America, South America and Europe, where statistics are the most detailed, the record of *new* cases (incidence) ranges from 2 to 8 per 1,000 each year. A study in Great Britain has calculated that up to 20,000 people might have lupus. Estimates in the USA range from 275,000 (women only) to a massive 1.7 million. This last figure comes from a survey commissioned by the Lupus Foundation of America and reported in 1994. It was obtained by ringing people and asking them if they had ever been told they have lupus. The researchers admit that estimating prevalence 'by unsubstantiated claim' yields a figure higher than previously expected. 'Self-reporting studies are notoriously inaccurate as the criteria for the disease are not verified, indicating that the numbers derived from this study may not be true.' Putting this extreme estimate on one side it is likely that the majority of available prevalence statistics conceal a lupus 'iceberg', with many more having the illness than get counted. However, national and global prevalence figures conceal really massive differences in distribution: between the sexes, between age, racial and socio-economic groups and, to some extent, according to where people live.

Gender

Ninety per cent of those who get lupus are women. (Some estimates put this even higher.) It is predominantly a disease that strikes women of childbearing years (see 'Age' below). This combination of characteristics suggests that vulnerability to lupus may be related to the reproductive hormone *oestrogen*. Men also get lupus, as do children and women beyond reproductive age, but in every age group or other grouping, women always outnumber men. In children, in whom hormonal effects are presumably minimal, for each male, 3 girls get lupus. In adults, the ratio ranges from 10 to 15 women for each man. In older people (women beyond the menopause when the production of reproductive hormones is reduced) the ratio is approximately 8 women for every man.

Age

As we have said: lupus strikes chiefly women during their reproductive years. Sixty-five per cent of patients first experience symptoms between the ages of 16 and 55. Of the remaining cases, 20 per cent are affected between 12 and 16 – by which age most women are sexually mature – and 15 per cent after the age of 55. Lupus does strike the very young and very old but not sufficiently to make a statistical contribution.

Race and geography

Different racial groups are more or less susceptible. This phenomenon is probably and principally related to the genetic differences between peoples. Tiny parts of the human *genome* – the information handed down from parent to child that programmes the growth and development of the body – vary from person to person and some genetic differences are more common in one race than another, making them differentially more or less prone to certain diseases.

There is more lupus among Afro-Caribbeans, Afro-Americans, Hispanic Americans, Asians and Asians living in the UK than among Caucasian people living in the same continents. In France, immigrants from Spain, Portugal, North Africa and Italy are more susceptible than native Frenchmen and women. In New Zealand both the prevalence and mortality of lupus are higher among Polynesians than Caucasians. The vulnerability of immigrant communities may be compounded by a general tendency for lupus to be more common in urban than rural communities.

This is a distinction lupus shares with rheumatoid arthritis. Africans living in Africa appear less susceptible, and certainly there is a general tendency for lupus to be more common among immigrants than in their homeland and in cooler rather than tropical climes. Some researchers have suggested that this could be because immigration nearly always involves a move to cooler climes from hotter ones, and that the reduction in the amount of sunlight could play a part (see Chapter 3).

Ethnic variables

In the 1990s the National Institution of Arthritis and Musculoskeletal and Skin Diseases (NIAMS), the agency in the USA concerned with rheumatic disorders, started recruiting several hundred lupus patients from various groups between the ages of 20 and 50, to take part in a study of all aspects of the disease, from clinical characteristics, through psychological factors and genetics and including the contribution of ethnic origin to the incidence of the disease. It's called LUMINA (see 'Useful addresses' at the end of this book), standing for LUpus in MInorities: NAture versus nurture, and at the moment it is still ongoing.

Is it serious, doctor?

Differences in disease severity and long-term outcome also occur between the different groups. For example, black or dark-skinned people – people originating in tropical countries – have a poorer

13

Lupus in history

The name 'lupus' for a skin disease has been around for more than seven centuries.

Thirteenth century The ancient Italian physician Rogerius describes a disease characterized by lesions which he calls 'lupus'. In medieval Latin the word for a wolf – lupus – was used to mean 'ulcerated', perhaps because sores or ulcers that eat into the face look rather like a wolf bite.

Seventeenth century Philosopher/physicians Paracelsus and Sennert provide clear descriptions of 'lupus' skin lesions.

1828 French dermatologist Laurent-Théodore Biett identifies three types of lupus and coins the term 'lupus erythemadoides' for the distinctive butterfly rash. His teachings are published this year by his pupil Pierre Cazenave in his *Practical summary of skin diseases* . . .

1873 Moritz Kaposi, professor of dermatology at the medical school at the University of Vienna, Austria, publishes a series of articles on lupus erythematosus, noting that patients with the rash also have other symptoms – in other words, that it is systemic; 'Lupus erythematosus . . . may be attended by altogether more severe pathological changes . . . and even dangerous constitutional symptoms may be intimately associated with the process in question, and that death may result from conditions which must be considered to arise from the local malady.'

1890 Thomas Payne, a physician at St Thomas' Hospital, London, is the first to recognize that anti-malarial drugs, long used to treat fever, may have more general healing powers for symptoms like joint pain and fatigue in lupus.

prognosis. Some studies also suggest that lupus is worse among those with less education, and those from lower socio-economic groups, though this may reflect the fact that such groups often have poorer access to health care or they may fail to follow treatment and health guidelines (known to doctors as poor *compliance*).

But these days, can lupus be fatal? Very rarely, is the short

1895–1903 In a series of papers the celebrated US physician William Osler describes other organs involved in lupus – heart, kidneys and other 'mucous surfaces' – and defines the condition as 'systemic' and also chronic: relapsing and remitting.

1941 On the basis of numerous post-mortem studies of damaged organs in lupus patients, Paul Klemperer, at the Mt Sinai Hospital, New York, proposes that lupus is a 'collagen vascular' disease. This term remains in use for fifty years or more.

1948 The diagnosis of lupus moves into a new phase: Malcolm Hargraves of the Mayo Clinic in Maryland, USA, identifies an odd-looking white blood cell, found first in the bone marrow, then in the blood of people with acute lupus. It becomes known as the LE (Lupus Erythematosus) cell. As a result, the first blood test for lupus is devised and the number of people diagnosed rises steadily.

1954–72 Over this period several other anomalies are detected in the blood of those with lupus. Chief of these is an antibody that works specifically against the body's own DNA (*deoxyribonucleic-acid* – the raw material of living systems). A test for this anti-nuclear antibody – ANA – replaces the LE as the gold-standard for detecting lupus, and lupus becomes located firmly in the family of autoimmune diseases. (Details of these sophisticated diagnostic tests are included in Chapter 4.)

1983 A group led by Graham Hughes at St Thomas' Hospital identifies the antibody associated with artery and vein thrombosis, strokes and miscarriages that had made pregnancy so risky for lupus sufferers; it is now known as the Hughes' syndrome. Treatment to counteract the effect of this *antiphospholipid antibody* is devised (more about this in Chapter 10).

answer. A 1955 survey showed a 5-year survival rate of only 50 per cent, but we now know that this dealt with a very small, seriously ill, largely untreated group of people with the disease. With today's broader picture, it is possible to say with some confidence that it is only rarely fatal. Survival rates are measured over 5, 10 and 20 years from diagnosis. In the mid-1990s survival at 5 and 10 years was nearer 95 per cent and even after 20 years it was over 85 per cent. If you have lupus now, with all the improvements in treatment available, it is highly unlikely to be life-threatening.

Lupus in young children

Lupus is rare in children under 12, the age around when girls usually start their periods. Below the age of 5 it is exceedingly rare, although specialist physicians see a small number of cases between that age and adolescence.

Very occasionally, newborn babies develop a lupus-like rash in the first weeks of life. This is not true lupus and only occurs because the mother has lupus and some of the antibodies that cause the disease have crossed the placenta from her blood into the baby's. As the maternal antibodies die down the rash also subsides. This condition is known as *neonatal* (newborn) lupus. (This is discussed in more detail in Chapter 10.)

Most authorities claim that there is essentially no difference in how lupus affects young children. They are a small group so that significant statistics are difficult to gather. However, some recent studies suggest their symptoms may often be more severe. A study from the European Working Party on Systemic Lupus Erythematosus found that the pattern of symptoms was different in young children and other minority subgroups: old people and men. Children were less likely to have *rheumatoid factor* (an antibody that is a frequent marker of inflammation in arthritis) in their bloodstream but more likely to suffer from the butterfly rash (also known as the *malar rash*), kidney problems, pericarditis and liver and blood complications. The rash or kidney problems were also the symptoms most likely to bring child lupus patients to the attention of a doctor.

Lupus in men

There are small differences in how lupus affects men compared with women. Men tend to be diagnosed at a later age, and the mortality rate one year after diagnosis (infinitesimally low in the treated population) is slightly higher. The study from the European Working Party on Systemic Lupus Erythematosus found that they were less likely to suffer from arthritis and photosensitivity than women, and that pleurisy and pericarditis were more frequently their presenting symptom – the one that made them consult a doctor – than for women with the disease.

Late-onset lupus in older people

In the context of lupus, 'older' is rather broadly interpreted by the statisticians as over 55: the age by which most women have passed the menopause. Notwithstanding this, and including men, some 15 per cent of lupus cases do not appear until this age. The European Working Party on Systemic Lupus Erythematosus found that at this age new patients were less likely to present with the butterfly rash, arthritis or kidney problems than children or younger people. These symptoms continued to feature less (about half as frequent) during the course of the illness, as did photosensitivity and thrombosis. However, they were twice as likely to suffer from dry eyes and mouth (*sicca syndrome*). Other studies found that the discoid rash – hard, raised plaques which sometimes leave scarring – was more common in patients who developed lupus late in their lives.

In developed countries, of course, older people are the most likely to be taking medication for all sorts of conditions other than lupus. This introduces a group of people who, independent of age and sex, develop lupus as a consequence of taking certain drugs. Known reasonably as 'drug-induced lupus' these are probably the only cases where the cause is emphatically certain and the cure obvious. The drug causing the problem has to be stopped or changed. (Drug-induced lupus is considered in more detail in Chapter 9.)

17

3
The causes of lupus – finding the wolf's lair

While no one knows what causes lupus, promising clues are scattered all over the place (like wolf prints outside a lair). Almost certainly there is no single cause, though we are able to rule some causes out:

- It is not transmitted by any infectious agent: bacterium, virus or parasite; so you can't 'catch' lupus from another person – though infection may play some part in sparking off lupus (more on this later).
- It is not caused by any known environmental agent: no industrial chemical, toxic fumes, inhaled fibres like asbestos, microwaves or radio masts – though again, some environmental agent may play a part in triggering the disease, or a flare-up.
- It is not, conversely, caused by a deficiency of anything – vitamin, essential mineral, vital nutrient, hormone or enzyme – needed during crucial stages of embryo or infant development.
- It does not represent an *allergic* reaction or sensitivity to anything sufferers (or their mothers) have eaten or been in contact with – though again, such factors may play a part in why some people develop lupus, and lupus sufferers are as likely to suffer allergies as anyone else.
- It is not caused by a gene, or genes, handed down from parent to child. This does not mean that there is not something in lupus sufferers' genetic inheritance that is making them more vulnerable to the disease.

Does it matter if we are unsure what causes lupus? Yes. You can treat an illness by using a mixture of experiment and observation, as ancient herbalists and witchdoctors knew, but you cannot hope to cure, let alone prevent it, unless you can understand the underlying causes of the disease. As knowledge of what goes wrong in the disease grows –invariably a complex chain reaction involving more than a single process in the body – doctors have more opportunities to intervene – a verb much in favour with medical scientists, making it possible to 'cut it off at the pass' and, ultimately, 'to stop it short in its tracks'.

So researchers are looking, not for a single cause, but for a combination of factors that lead to a person developing lupus.

A genetic predisposition?

While lupus is not caused by a defective gene handed down from mother to child, there is certainly evidence that some genetic factor is at work. When lupus is diagnosed it is not uncommon to find that there are relatives who have had lupus or at the very least lupus-like symptoms. What seems likely is that some genetic vulnerability to developing the disease is inherited, though not the disease itself. A child with lupus in the family may be born a lupus 'sleeper', the vulnerability gene lying dormant until sparked into action by some trigger in the outside world.

Ginny's story
While she was in her mid-twenties Ginny's husband Bob was posted to East Africa with the RAF and she went with him. She had always been an outdoor person and in Nairobi she was able to swim and ride and spend from dawn to the equatorial dusk in the open. When she first noticed the rash on her face she thought perhaps she had caught a touch of the sun, though she tanned easily and had never before been bothered with sunburn. She wore a hat and slapped on protective cream for a while and it seemed to clear up. Then the aches and pains in her hands started. She didn't have the energy or inclination to go riding or to the swimming pool. The unit medical officer murmured something about 'arthritis' and suggested aspirin. Ginny suffered silently indoors. In her weekly international phone call home she complained of her painful hands to her mum. Her mum said, 'I think you could have lupus.' Ginny's aunt had nearly died during her first pregnancy, she said, and had been diagnosed as having lupus. 'Come to think of it, you used to complain of pains in your hands and wrists after playing tennis when you were at school', said her mother. 'We just put it down to growing pains.'

Will my baby get it?

Remember 'growing pains'. They crop up again in Chapter 4. Experienced rheumatologists have commented on how often they are mentioned in the history of people with lupus diagnosed after they have grown up.

When a woman develops lupus she learns that she may have problems with pregnancy. After asking 'Is it all right to have children?' she will almost certainly ask, 'Will my baby get lupus?' While there is a slightly increased chance of this – about 5 per cent – at least the baby of a lupus mother is unlikely to develop lupus unnoticed. As explained, lupus belongs to the autoimmune family of diseases and there is a great deal of overlap in how the immune system malfunctions and the symptoms that result from such diseases. Support for the idea that there is some inherited predisposition to develop autoimmune disease comes from several directions. First, the relations of those with autoimmune conditions are more likely to have the same or a similar condition. About 20 per cent of lupus sufferers have first-degree relatives – parent, child or sibling – who have either lupus or some other autoimmune condition like insulin-dependent diabetes or rheumatoid arthritis. What's more, if the blood of a lupus sufferer's healthy close relatives is tested a further 20 per cent are found to carry immunological oddities characteristic of people with lupus, although at the time they show no outward signs of disease. These relatives may be the 'sleepers' who have inherited a susceptibility gene which has so far not been triggered and become active

Twin studies

Comparing identical twins is the ideal way to quantify the genetic contribution to the development of a condition. Identical twins are made of identical genetic material: they share the same DNA – the basic building blocks that programme living systems. If twins share a characteristic, like blue eyes or a musical ear, they are said to be *concordant.* If they differ they are said to be *dis*cordant. Identical twins start out with a high level of concordance just because they are formed from the same egg and the same DNA. If they are brought up together they also share the same environment so their concordance is increased. Fraternal twins do not come from the same egg; they are only as alike as two siblings, although born at the same time. But they will share their environment if brought up together.

The likelihood that fraternal twins will be concordant for lupus is no more than it is for siblings born at different times – a mere 2 to 5 per cent. But identical twins have a much higher concordance; various studies estimate it to be from 24 per cent to as high as 57 per cent. From the point of view of quantifying the genetic component in developing lupus the interesting thing is why it is no more than 57 per cent. These children share not only genes, they share environment during childhood. What happened differently to the one who developed lupus, which didn't touch his or her sibling? A gene for susceptibility may have been inherited, but it is clearly not the whole story.

Twin studies: the latest

In 2003, to increase our understanding of the role of genetic inheritance in developing autoimmune diseases, the National Institution of Environmental Health Science in the USA launched a search for same-sex siblings – twins or close-in-age brother or sister pairs – where one sibling had an autoimmune disease but the other did not. (By selecting same-sex, close-in-age pairs the variability conferred by age and sex differences is eliminated from the study.) They plan to enrol 400 pairs, which may take a while for such a select grouping, but they hope that this research will give clearer answers to the role of genes that predispose susceptible individuals to whatever triggers autoimmune diseases (see Chapter 11).

X marks the vulnerable spot

Before we leave the genetic connection there is another inherited component that appears to affect who succumbs to the bite of the wolf and who escapes.

About thirty years ago when the first transplants took place, medical interest became focused upon why and how transplants from a donor were rejected by the recipient's body. How did each individual body distinguish between 'self' and 'foreign' and fight the foreign invader as vigorously and efficiently as if it had been a splinter, or a boil? They discovered that every human cell carries an inherited code that controls a number of immune responses including the acceptance or rejection of transplanted tissue and organs.

Everyone belongs to one or another *major histocompatibility complex* (*histos* is the Greek word for tissue), or MHC, just as all of us belong to one of several blood groups that determine what type of donor blood is acceptable for transfusion. If a recipient is in the same MHC as the donor then the transplant will not be perceived as 'foreign' by the immune system and has a better chance of being accepted by the body. Scientists can now pick up markers for people's MHC from their blood just as they are able to read their blood group. These are called *antigens,* because they generate 'anti' behaviour towards an invader – germs or transplanted tissue. They also identify people who may be susceptible to certain diseases.

In the early 1970s an MHC marker was identified in 80 per cent of those with the dauntingly named *ankylosing spondylitis* – a disabling form of spinal arthritis, which strikes mostly men and had been observed to run in families. The marker was found in only 10 per cent of people without the disease. Since then MHC markers linked to several other diseases have been found; rheumatoid arthritis, insulin-dependent diabetes and, yes, lupus. All these are autoimmune conditions so perhaps it is not surprising that shared inherited factors that affect the operation of the immune system should be common to so many people with these diseases.

Since you inherit your MHC from your parents and grandparents the same groups tend to run in families. This is why brothers, sisters or even more distant relations are sought whenever someone needs a transplant of bone marrow. By the same reasoning certain MHCs will be more common in one ethnic group than another, which goes some way to explain why certain racial groups or nationalities may have a higher incidence of some diseases.

Markers for MHCs are not the only clues to understanding lupus that can be detected from tests on the patient's blood (see Chapter 4 for more details of these).

'Sometimes it's hard to be a woman'

Since nine times as many women as men get lupus surely it seems obvious that femaleness must be to blame? Women have two X chromosomes and men have one X and one Y. Could there be something on that second X chromosome that makes women more vulnerable to lupus than men? Or could something on the male Y chromosome be protecting them? A genetic disease like *haemophilia* works exactly like this: it is carried on one X chromosome but in the presence of a second X lies dormant. So women carry the disease but never exhibit the bleeding disorder. However, if a man inherits the defective X chromosome he only has just the one and his Y chromosome doesn't suppress the illness. He bleeds.

We know that it doesn't work like this for lupus or the differences between the sexes would be much more dramatic and the concordance of twins would be absolute.

So if not chromosomes what about hormones? Aren't they part of what makes men and women different? We know that the highest concentration of women developing the disease coincides with their reproductive years when the sex hormones are most active. One major hospital study of all the children and teenagers developing lupus over a period of ten years found that a substantial spurt of new cases occurred at the ages of eleven and twelve, the age of puberty.

But if female hormones were responsible for this dramatic phenomenon, you would expect the balance of hormones in those who develop lupus to be noticeably different from those who do not. (It is the balance between hormones that counts rather than absolute levels.) Certainly female hormones (*oestrogens*) were found to aggravate the symptoms of laboratory mice with a lupus-like illness, and male hormones (*androgens*) appeared to protect them. However, making an existing illness worse or better is not the same as causing it, and something that protects or cures mice might not work for humans.

Studies of assorted male and female hormone levels in humans with lupus are mostly inconclusive. Sometimes they are higher than average; sometimes lower but not consistently so. An additional problem is that normal men and women both carry the same hormones; it is the balance between them that distinguishes the sexes. A significantly lower-than-average level of one hormone *was* found in both men and women. This was a form of androgen called *dehydroepiandrosterone (DHEA)*, which is a precursor of both the male hormone testosterone and the female hormones oestradiol and progesterone. (The fluctuating balance of these two regulates fertility in women.) If something is in short supply it is always possible that raising it will produce an improvement or confer protection, as it did for the lab mice, so the role of DHEA is one avenue that is being investigated. Abnormal levels of another hormone, prolactin – which in women plays a major role in enabling the production of breast milk – is being investigated in both men and women. (See Chapter 11 for drugs that affect these hormones.)

It's not what you've got, it's what you do with it that counts

But before we finish with hormones as a possible cause of lupus susceptibility, let us look at what happens to them in the body. Perhaps it is not the levels, or even the balance of hormones that makes lupus sufferers different; perhaps it is how their bodies *metabolize* them – break them down and put them to use. Several other conditions are caused by a failure to metabolize something useful rather than a shortage of the raw material itself. For example, type 2 diabetes is caused, not by underproduction of insulin as is type 1, but by the failure of the body to utilize the hormone. Other diseases are caused by the inability to break down and absorb the foods that contain essential nutrients even when the diet itself is not deficient. After the menopause, reduced levels of oestrogens make it more difficult for women to absorb calcium, even if they maintain a diet rich in the chemical, and this increases the risk of *osteoporosis* – brittle, easily broken bones (see Chapter 7).

Some studies have indeed found that patients of both sexes with lupus metabolized oestrogens differently from other people (the hormones that aggravated lupus in mice). This is an avenue researchers are continuing to explore.

Environmental triggers and the infection connection

Why then does one identical twin develop lupus while the other doesn't, given that both share the same genetic vulnerability and MHC? The prevailing idea is that something in the environment triggers the disease, but since both twins are susceptible it figures that only one can have been exposed to the crucial trigger.

The most popular candidate for an environmental trigger is infection early in life. This theory is proposed for a number of diseases where the autoimmune system starts attacking the body's own tissues. The hypothesis is that, faced with an infection, the immune system very properly gets to work to fight it, but for some

24

reason when the infection is vanquished, instead of withdrawing, the immune system turns its guns on healthy tissue. This could be what happens in insulin-dependent diabetes, in leukaemia and in rheumatoid arthritis; some quite unremarked infection flicks the switch and starts the antibodies off in the wrong direction.

The infectious agents that best fit the profile of a lupus trigger are viruses. Viruses are cellular parasites, definitely not nice to know. There are many varieties and what they all have in common is that they break into a living cell, hijack its reproductive system to make little virus offspring and lurk, concealed in the body, sometimes for years. Because they hide inside cells it makes it very difficult for the immune system to access and destroy them. Nevertheless the body usually manages to generate antibodies against a virus. The presence of such antibodies in the blood of a patient therefore becomes like the footprint of where a virus has been even when the symptoms of an acute attack have gone.

Researchers hot on the trail of a lupus trigger have looked for antibodies that might reveal that particular viruses have been there. Two studies, one in France the other in the USA, thought they detected antibodies to a retrovirus, but were unable to link it to any known human variety like HIV. Other researchers have looked for signs that infection by one of the *herpesviruses* might be responsible for triggering lupus, or other autoimmune diseases. Herpes, as explained in the 'Know your virus' box overleaf, stays dormant in the body once it has invaded it, but it only flares up – rather like lupus – occasionally, usually when the body is under stress.

The evidence from these studies is encouraging – some patients with lupus, and related autoimmune disorders, did indeed appear to have elevated levels of antibodies to some of the viruses considered. But there again, these are pretty common viruses; many people have been exposed to them, so there is nothing very solid proved against them yet.

Nevertheless experts are confident they are looking in the right place for a lupus trigger in targeting viruses. Sheldon Blau says:

It is likely when the primary cause of lupus is found – and it *will* be found eventually – it will turn out to be a virus, whether a retrovirus, a herpesvirus or some other type that behaves in an unusual manner (or is permitted to behave in an unusual manner in some individuals, perhaps those with particular genetic characteristics).

Know your virus

There are many groups and subdivisions of viruses. Viruses are composed of an inner core of genetic material – the bit that reproduces itself – surrounded by a coat of protein. (In diagrams they look a bit like a chestnut or a sea mine, with a spiky outer layer.) The genetic core may be made of either DNA (the material that we are made of) or a slight variation called *ribonucleic acid* (*RNA*).

The DNA group includes a large family of viruses responsible for many childhood nose, throat and eye infections. The bad relations in this clan are the poxvirus, which is responsible for smallpox, the milder cowpox, from which smallpox vaccines are made, and the notorious herpesviruses. The name, herpes, comes from the Latin and Greek for 'creep' and is also used for a reptile or serpent. Various members of the herpesvirus tribe cause cold sores, genital sores, chicken-pox and shingles – where the blisters or lesions 'creep' round the body. Once they have got you, you have them for life. Herpesviruses are being investigated as candidates for a lupus trigger.

The RNA family of viruses also includes both troublesome children and wicked uncles. The members of one group make themselves at home in the mucous lining of the nose and throat, and are called myxoviruses (*myxa* is Greek for mucus). Influenza is a myxovirus. Their close relations, the paramyxoviruses, include measles, mumps and scarlet fever and there is also a parainfluenza virus that causes coughs and colds. (The Greek prefix *para* means

And Blau advances yet another interesting hypothesis. Could the autoimmune illnesses like lupus be triggered in people with the genetic susceptibility because they are subject to attack from *two or more* directions at the same time? 'Perhaps the massive autoreactive activity in these conditions stems from a frenzied immune-system effort to stave off simultaneous acute infections by, say, a retrovirus *and* a herpesvirus.'

The wolf's domestic cousins – pets

Viruses are not the only suspects in the search for a lupus trigger in the environment. There is a particular group of people more prone to beside or closely related to.) Another group which is worth remembering is the retroviruses – a group you will hear a lot about. For some time it had been known that retroviruses caused illness in animals. Then in 1981 a retrovirus was found to be the cause of a rare form of human leukaemia which damaged a group of cells that are part of the immune system called T-*lymphocytes*. This retrovirus was christened 'human T-cell lymphotropic virus', or HTLV for short. Later another similar retrovirus was identified – HTLV-2 – and still later another – HTLV-3. This last became perhaps the most celebrated and feared retrovirus in history. It is now better known as the human immunodeficiency virus – HIV. Over a period of years it wreaks such havoc in the immune system that, untreated, it leads to death from AIDS.

But back to lymphocytes. In addition to T-lymphocytes – the ones implicated in the rare leukaemia and HIV – there are also B kinds. When a foreign invader is detected, B-lymphocytes produce antibodies specifically to attack that particular invader (they are antigen-specific). Two types of T-lymphocyte work along side these B cells. T 'helper' cells do exactly what the name implies and support the work of B cells, partly by cleaning up the debris of the battle against foreign invaders. T 'suppressor' cells do just the opposite. They act like a damper or prefect, to make sure B cells don't get overenthusiastic in their activity. The T suppressor cells fail to do their job in several autoimmune diseases.

lupus and other autoimmune disorders that we haven't mentioned so far: pet owners.

By and large diseases do not jump species. (There are some infamous exceptions like swine flu and the recent cases of new-variant CJD contracted from diseased cattle; and children often catch the fungal infection ringworm from their pets.)

The wolf's domestic cousin, the pet dog, is implicated. The fact that dogs develop lupus became widely known in the USA when, in the early 1990s, President George Bush senior and his wife Barbara both developed a condition called Graves' disease, an autoimmune disease of the thyroid gland. At the same time it was discovered that the Bushes' dog Millie had lupus.

Tess's story

Tess developed lupus while doing her finals at university. Her family had been watching anxiously for the illness ever since Tess had started her periods because her mother also had lupus and she had discovered the illness during the 1950s when she had become pregnant and then lost her first child. In spite of everything, Tess managed to complete her finals and, once she started taking an antimalarial drug, the rash that had sprung up on her face and down her back, her arms and on her chest began to calm down. During the summer holidays she relaxed, took it easy and it looked as though the first flare was behind her. And then she noticed a funny thing. Her cat Jinxy was off her food. She stayed on her cushion reluctant to move and, when she did, appeared to be stiff and in pain. Tess took Jinxy to the vet and he discovered that she had quite severe ulcers in her mouth. 'Stomatitis' he called it. But Tess was convinced her cat had lupus. 'Cats don't get lupus', insisted the vet, but he agreed to give Jinxy a corticosteroid injection and, within a few days, she appeared to get better.

Unusual anecdotes do not constitute proof. However, where dogs are concerned there is solid evidence that they do suffer from a form of lupus, exhibiting symptoms similar to humans – arthritis, skin lesions (mostly around the nose) aggravated by sunlight, and kidney problems – with a similar pattern of flare-up and remission and responsive to the same drugs. So could there be transmission between pet and owner? A small study published in *The Lancet* in 1992 offers some support to this notion. A group of dogs owned by patients with lupus was compared with an outwardly healthy group owned by non-sufferers, and also with a group of dogs diagnosed as already having lupus. To all outward appearances the lupus-owners' dogs were perfectly healthy, but when their blood was tested it was found to have significantly higher levels of the antibodies characteristic of lupus sufferers' blood than were found in both the healthy control animals, and even the dogs known to have lupus! Something linked the lupus humans and their dogs, but what exactly? A link between pet ownership and a higher incidence of other autoimmune diseases has also been found, though not always supported by blood tests that demonstrate that pets and owners carry the same antibodies.

28

Scientists are always reminding us that because two things happen at the same time, or follow each other, it doesn't mean that one *causes* the other. It could be coincidence. It could be that both events share a common cause; some environmental trigger or infectious agent which affects pets and humans that live together. One thing is certain however: pets and human owners don't share the same genetic susceptibility!

Other possible environmental triggers

One or two other possible lupus triggers have been investigated.

Smoking is known to trigger a flare-up in people with lupus. A number of recent studies point to smokers being as much as two times more susceptible to lupus as non-smokers. A similar effect has been noted with other autoimmune diseases.

Evidence that an environmental pollutant is contributing to an illness is usually found in the form of *clusters*: that is, an increased incidence of a disease in particular localities or geographical areas. Clusters of juvenile leukaemia were discovered in areas around the nuclear power plant in Sellafield in Cumbria, suggesting that the plant was in some way triggering the illness. Pesticides and some industrial toxins have been implicated in other diseases. Lupus clusters are very rare. One was reported in Arizona in the mid-1990s, and exposure to pesticides or other industrial contaminants was postulated as a possible cause, but not backed up by firm evidence.

A number of therapeutic drugs are also known to cause lupus or, more correctly, lupus-like symptoms. It's not true lupus because, once the drugs are withdrawn, the condition disappears and does not recur (more about drug-induced lupus in Chapter 9).

This has been a long chapter because, given the uncertainty surrounding the disease, it has been necessary to consider many factors in order to explore its possible causes. When the various steps that lead to lupus are eventually understood a much shorter chapter will be required – though longer chapters may then have to be written on treating, curing or even preventing lupus!

4

Diagnosing lupus – on the trail of the wolf 1: in the surgery

For the patients the experience of lupus starts with symptoms: how they feel and what they see – the rash, the aches and pains, the hair on the comb, the fatigue. The doctor also is first presented with the patient's symptoms: some can be seen, others discovered by asking questions – taking a history – and others discovered through the doctor's knowledge of how the healthy body works and what signs indicate things are going wrong.

Unless faced with the classic butterfly rash, few GPs are likely to diagnose lupus 'at the surgery door'. Even with painstaking history-taking and examination (the first two parts of diagnosis), certainty may evade them. The frequency with which fatigue, depression or general aches and pains are the first presenting symptoms easily deceives the primary-care physician and although there is now a battery of laboratory tests which have revolutionized the diagnosis of lupus, a doctor needs to know which tests to order.

Lupus patients often see several doctors before they are correctly diagnosed. In 2002 the American Autoimmune Related Diseases Association reported that the majority of those with serious autoimmune diseases had had difficulty in obtaining a diagnosis. Many had been told their symptoms were 'in their heads' or that they were suffering from stress. No fewer than 45 per cent had been told they were hypochondriacs! A wise GP may order some of the basic tests as soon as he or she has seen the patient, but will also refer the person to a specialist rheumatology department.

Taking a history

Here, the person details her symptoms to the doctor, and the doctor asks questions, to gain maximum information. The aim is to narrow down the possible explanations – disease candidates – and then to eliminate them and arrive at a differential diagnosis. Suppose the patient has fatigue, fever, a rash, hair loss or aches and pains; the

30

doctor needs to rule out: infection, some allergic reaction or a hormonal imbalance, to name just a few conditions that might cause similar symptoms. Suppose the doctor advances to the conclusion that the patient has some autoimmune condition, or indeed one of the connective tissue diseases? He or she is still only at first base. How can the field be reduced to one?

To make this task easier, the American College of Rheumatology (ACR) publishes a list of diagnostic criteria for each of the connective tissue disorders. These are basically tick-boxes of symptoms and signs that have been found to accompany confirmed diagnosis of each condition in international studies of disease. They are not a substitute for the individual doctor's examination of the individual patient but they provide guidelines on what should be covered in an examination, and ensure that it is as thorough as possible. ACR's diagnostic criteria for lupus were first drawn up thirty years ago and have been revised several times. The important physical symptoms listed are familiar. Some are more significant than others because they are highly specific to lupus (see the box 'Specificity and sensitivity' on p. 34). Taken all together they build up a composite picture.

ACR symptoms detected in the surgery

- **Butterfly (malar) rash** – the oft-cited 'classic' symptom – 'probably more due to its picturesque name than its prevalence', says Sheldon Blau. The rash may not be itchy or painful, but may burn slightly on exposure to sunlight. It usually disappears leaving no mark.
- **Discoid lesions** – these are the circular raised, red, scaly plaques more common in men and first-time, older lupus patients, which were once considered a separate form of the disease because they are often the only lupus symptom patients have. These lesions can leave scarring and permanent hair loss when they heal.
- **Photosensitivity of the skin** – this rash specifically follows exposure to sunlight or fluorescent light. Although it occurs in no more than a third of lupus patients it is often a presenting symptom and it is highly specific to lupus, particularly if it is accompanied by lupus-type symptoms in other parts of the body (see box 'Specificity and sensitivity' on p. 34).

Diagnosis: craft or science?

Diagnosis, doctors are taught, is like Gaul – divided into three parts: you take a history from the patient; you examine; you do tests. You then collate and compare this information with the features of diseases known to you in the hope of making a match or at the very least a differential diagnosis: 'It can't be this, this or this; so, by elimination, it must be that.' In practice doctors hardly ever work like this.

Doctors are fond of joking to each other that they can diagnose their patients 'at the surgery door'. And of course, much of what family doctors see is the same – coughs, colds, stress, domestic battle-fatigue and old age – but it is also because they become practised in reading their patients' ills from subtle signs. In the words of one doctor, 'The eye of the experienced beholder is worth a laboratory-load of tests.' This diagnosis by intuition or divination conjures up the old idea of the doctor as magical, medicine man, though in practice it is actually diagnosis by expertise gained through experience. The Oxford Handbook of Clinical Medicine (OHCM) calls divination diagnosis 'diagnosis by recognition' and it probably applies less to lupus than to other conditions; nevertheless it is interesting to consider this and the other styles of diagnosis in outline.

Diagnosis by recognition

This is 'surgery door' diagnosis that comes with years of experience. It impresses both patient and student (when present). It is hard to quantify and harder still to teach, and it is not infallible. The OHCM says 20 per cent of such diagnoses are demonstrably wrong. Fortunately, the modern laboratory detects such error.

Diagnosis by reasoning

This is the Sherlock Holmes technique. The evidence for and against each candidate disease is considered, with the aim of excluding it. Whatever remains after elimination is the diagnosis,

• **Ulcerative sores** – these blister-like sores are sometimes, but not always, painless and affect the mucous lining of the mouth and throat, and occasionally the vagina. If painless, a dentist may pick them up before the patient.

however unlikely. This system fails because the list of candidates may not include the actual illness in the first place, or because the reasons for dismissing some candidates are faulty. This is why it belongs, like Holmes, in fiction, says OHCM.

Diagnosis by Wait on Events (WoE)

This was a popular diagnostic technique in the distant past when there was little doctors could do to treat or cure, so that inaction was in many cases less harmful than action that might turn out to be wrong. A celebrated doctor observed that, of the patients who came to his consulting room, 50 per cent would get better whatever he did, 25 per cent would get worse whatever he did, and 25 per cent might actually benefit from what he could do. The advantage of WoE was that he reduced the people needing help by the half who recovered, and his success rate doubled to 50 per cent of the remainder. Of course it's not as simple as that, but WoE still often figures in a modern doctor's notes. Even in chronic conditions like lupus, a pattern, or an additional confirmatory symptom, may appear while you are waiting for those all-important laboratory tests.

Diagnosis by hypothesis

This is the classic scientist's approach, not unlike Sherlock Holmes'. Postulate a diagnosis and then try and disprove it. It's thorough, but lengthy, so in some way not unlike WoE. Something will probably happen to the patient that illuminates things while the doctor is hypothesizing.

Diagnosis by computer

This increasingly popular technique is as new as WoE is old. It has its advantages: the computer gives access to a range of expertise in addition to the doctor's own. It may throw up some curious options – the computer can't see the patient coming through the surgery door – but among them may be something the doctor hadn't thought of.

- **Arthritis** – pain in motion, stiffness, tenderness and swelling of peripheral (hands arms, feet and legs) joints caused by inflammation is the other classic symptom of lupus. Three-quarters of lupus patients present with it and 90 per cent suffer from it at some

33

Sensitivity and specificity

Laboratory tests supplement the physician's know-how and intuition, but they are still far from perfect. And they are imperfect in two different ways that also apply to clinical signs. First they identify *some* but not *all* who have a disease – that is, they sometimes give a false negative result; or, second, they give a positive result for some people *without* the disease – a false positive. If the test picks out say 99 of every 100 people with the disease it is said to be extremely sensitive. If it only gives one false positive result for every 100 people *without* the disease it is said to be extremely specific.

So does it matter? Surely 99 per cent accuracy is pretty good? Think of it like this: you are a guard with an X-ray gun which enables you to see if anyone coming through a checkpoint is carrying a hidden bomb. If the test for a hidden bomb is positive you blow the terrorist to kingdom come. If the X-ray gun sees nothing, the traveller is an innocent tourist whom you let pass with a wave. Now suppose your X-ray gun shows a shadow just like a hidden bomb and you blow it up and – oops, it was a harmless tourist carrying a cine-camera! Or suppose your X-ray gun misses a terrorist with a bomb and he gets through undetected. Just as bad. So it is with false negatives and false positives for disease. It is not too serious with a disease like lupus, but suppose you get a false negative for HIV? That person may go on to spread the life-threatening disease unaware of being at risk. And if you give someone a false positive for HIV a life will be blighted even though that person may not have the disease. This is why so much store is set by the sensitivity and specificity of tests, and it is unusual to rely upon just one test. As with clinical signs, wherever possible several different tests are used, and if results are negative the tests may be repeated, just in case they were false.

time, but although common, this symptom is by no means specific to lupus. Literally hundreds of conditions cause joint pain and it is at the top of the list of symptoms seen by GPs. At first meeting it is indistinguishable from rheumatoid arthritis. Subsequent laboratory tests sort one cause from another.

- **Chest/heart problems** – the most common of these is pleurisy: inflammation of the membrane enclosing the lungs. But patients may also have pericarditis: inflammation of the membrane surrounding the heart. The patient usually complains of chest pain especially when breathing deeply. Like arthritis this is not a symptom in any way specific to lupus, and a GP will first wish to exclude acute causes like infection or cancer. Again laboratory tests help sort one cause from another.

- **Kidney disorder** – the kidneys are sometimes known as the 'silent' organs in lupus because inflamed kidneys produce no obvious symptoms for patient or doctor. (Pain around the kidneys is more likely to be caused by something completely different: a urinary-tract infection or a kidney stone.) The clearest evidence that the kidneys are in trouble is fragments of protein or blood cells leaking into the urine that make it look cloudy. Healthy kidneys filter out protein and blood, and the urine is clear and sterile. Another sign that the kidneys may be inflamed is raised blood pressure. Testing blood pressure and urine is a standard part of a thorough medical examination, so GPs will usually pick up any kidney involvement. Some half of all lupus patients may have a degree of kidney involvement at some time; reports vary. Once again, taken alone, kidney problems are not specific to lupus.

- **Signs of neurological disorder** – lupus affects blood vessels all over the body. Inflammation of those in the brain may cause headaches, severe migraines with flashing lights, nausea or vomiting, or even alarming symptoms like seizures or signs of mental disturbance: exaggerated and irrational fears (phobias) or hallucinations. These brain symptoms have only recently been recognized as indicative of lupus and in the past some patients were diagnosed as having schizophrenia. But the accumulation of symptoms in other parts of the body confirms their underlying inflammatory origins.

Faced with a long row of ticks against these clinical signs a GP would treat the presenting symptoms but also refer the patient to a specialist rheumatologist, while ordering some laboratory tests that would help confirm his or her provisional diagnosis of lupus. These are explored in the next chapter.

5

Diagnosing lupus – on the trail of the wolf 2: in the laboratory

Around a hundred amd fifty years ago, observed or 'clinical' symptoms, as described in the last chapter, were all the doctor had to go on and they were not usually conclusive. These days, doctors can call up a raft of sophisticated laboratory tests. Blood or another sample may be taken in the surgery, but the analysis is completed by machines and skilled technicians in the pathology laboratory. Advanced and expensive imaging technology which reveals details inaccessible to the human eye is also available. It makes you realize why GPs often complain they are just a staging-post in modern medicine.

The American College of Rheumatology (ACR) diagnostic criteria include important evidence which can't be detected at a primary-care consultation, but require laboratory tests. Up to this point it has been sufficient for us to say that most lupus symptoms are caused by inflammation – inflammation prompted by an unexplained malfunction of the immune system. But if we are to go further and explain how the disease is detected in the laboratory we need to look at the inflammatory process and its causes in more detail.

Inflammation: the good news and the bad

Inflammation feels the same wherever it occurs – a sore throat, a splinter, a corn or arthritic joints: warmth, redness, swelling and pain. The amount of inflammation, hence the severity of the symptoms, is usually proportional to the severity of the injury or infection.

The body is a self-maintaining, self-repairing organism. Inflammation, though it may feel unpleasant, is actually a signal that the attack/defend/repair armoury of the immune system is at work. There are a number of weapons in this armoury – WMD: weapons of microscopic destruction, if you wish – each of which has a slightly different role to play in co-ordinating attack and in returning the immune system to normal afterwards. White cells or lymphocytes (the name indicates cells produced in the *lymph* glands, among other places) are the foot soldiers of inflammation. They are sub-divided into B cells and T cells. The T cells have their own role in fighting viruses and tumours, and also influence the behaviour of B cells.

At the start of an attack B cells produce antibodies specifically tailored to repel the invader. 'Helper' T cells assist, and there are back-up troops called *complement* – they complement the activity of antibodies in neutralizing the antigen. The embattled cluster of warring antigen, antibody and complement is called an *immune complex*. If you think of it like a rugby scrum, or a knot of heavies in a bar-room brawl, you can see why inflammation causes so much damage to surrounding tissues, particularly the kidneys in lupus: the equivalent of broken glass, splintered furniture and torn curtains. The objective is to destroy the antigen, but a lot more gets damaged in the process. During the battle, damaged cells at the site of infection or injury send out alarm-calls in the form of chemical messengers called *cytokines* to summon the foot soldiers. (There are many different forms of these chemical messengers active in inflammation: some put out the call to battle; others tell the troops to back off when the enemy is vanquished.) T 'suppressor' cells come onto the scene later to tell the B cells to back off when their work is done (more of them later).

While the inflammation rages, the blood supply to the battlefield is increased, producing redness and warmth, and the body's temperature rises. Clear fluid and white cells pass through the walls of the blood vessels into the surrounding tissues, causing swelling and pain as a result of the pressure upon the surrounding tissues. While the fluid dilutes poisons and is mildly antiseptic the white cells engulf, break down and remove any foreign particles like bacteria that they encounter, cleaning up the battlefield so that reconstruction can begin. The fluid – called inflammatory exudate – has the same capacity as blood to clot, and it will seal off clean wounds, like those resulting from a surgical operation or minor infection. The clot sticks the edges of the wound together so that new tissue can grow to heal the breach.

If the enemy is not swiftly routed, pus may form, composed of inflammatory exudate and broken-down cells of dead bacteria and white cells. (You may need to blow your nose, clear your throat, or lance an abscess.) The bone marrow and other blood-forming tissues are stimulated to produce yet more white cells. Ultimately, in the normal course of events, inflammation is self-limiting: T suppressors call a halt once the infection is cleared or the wound healed. However, in autoimmune diseases like lupus and rheumatoid arthritis 'it ain't necessarily so'.

Immune system malfunction

Autoimmune diseases affect players in the immune system. For example, in AIDS the virus attacks T helper cells and they become depleted so that people with the disease eventually succumb to a range of opportunistic infections which a healthy immune system would normally take in its stride. In lupus, as in rheumatoid arthritis, the problem is an overactive immune system. The antibody-producing B cells increase eight- to tenfold and the T suppressor cells, designed to suppress antibody production once the alien invader has been vanquished, are in short supply. B cells that produce antibodies with no obvious enemy to attack are called *autoreactive* – in other words, reacting to the body itself – and one of the things they appear to attack is immature T suppressor cells, which may explain the shortage of mature active ones in people with lupus.

A healthy immune system, like other body systems, depends on balance; on the right number of actors playing their part at the right time, delivering the right lines, and then leaving the stage. For more than thirty years scientists have known that lupus B cells continue to produce antibodies when there is nothing to attack and have been trying to fathom why. Is it that they are still getting messages (via those important cytokines) to attack, or are they failing to get the message (other important cytokines) to stop? And is that because too many 'Attack!' messages go out, or too few 'Back off!' messages? Is the problem too many or too few message-senders – helper T cells or suppressor T cells – or is it that the right messages get scrambled and don't get through to the overactive B cells? When you realize how complex the interaction of these immune-system actors is you can see how difficult it is to unravel which passage in the play has gone wrong. From the point of view of scientists trying to put things right it means lots of different places where they can try to intervene (that favourite verb again).

There is a colourful cartoon version of the inflammation

battleground plus what goes wrong in lupus on the University of Alabama's website (see 'Useful addresses' for the web address).

Messages in blood

From the point of view of the doctors trying to make a diagnosis it means that there are lots of potentially malfunctioning components to look for in the lupus patient's blood. The blood is the transport system of the body and a great deal of information can be obtained by unpacking the things carried around the body in the bloodstream at any one time. Other bodily functions are also informative: urine, the fluid inside joints or the spinal cord, blood-pressure readings and recordings of the electrical activity of the heart and brain. But in lupus blood tests are vital. So if you have it, resign yourself to having a lot of needles stuck into you.

The remainder of the ACR diagnostic criteria for lupus are detected from blood tests.

- **Haematological (blood) abnormalities.** These usually show up in a complete blood count (CBC), a procedure as basic as taking a pulse or blood-pressure measurement. Almost all lupus patients will have some abnormal factor in their blood at some time in their illness. There could be a shortage of red blood cells, the ones that carry oxygen round the body, called *erythrocytes* (Greek for 'red cells'). Shortage of red blood cells is called anaemia (the names for things in blood often end in *-aemia*, from the Greek for 'blood'). Or there may be a shortage of white cells (the ones that fight disease), called leucopoenia (Greek for 'white' and 'deficit'), or there could be a shortage of blood-clotting cells called *platelets* or *thrombocytes* (Greek for 'clotting cells'); this leads to excessive bleeding, either in the form of bruises or the bursting of small blood vessels in the skin, or sometimes the failure of a wound to heal properly. Doctors also test the rate at which red cells in unclotted blood form sediment at the bottom of a test tube: a simple, non-specific test called the *erythrocyte sedimentation rate (ESR)*. If there is inflammation or raised autoimmune activity in the body, the cells break down and the sediment collects more rapidly. It's simple but rather crude, with several limitations. For example, sedimentation may speed up for all sorts of reasons:

because the patient has an infection or from any number of inflammatory conditions other than lupus; and indeed patients can be quite ill but have a normal ESR. Then again, it slows down if the patient is taking certain common drugs, like penicillin, diuretics or vitamin A. But a doctor who has taken a thorough history will be alerted to this complication. Blood may also be tested for C-reactive protein (CRP), which is produced by the liver in response to inflammation. Like ESR the presence of CRP is an indicator of acute inflammation, though not specifically for lupus. It is more sensitive than ESR because it is only rarely found to be abnormally high in the blood of healthy people. Both ESR and CRP are useful when it comes to monitoring the success or otherwise of treatment.

- **Immunological disruption.** As we explained, in lupus there is a massive increase in the number of antibodies circulating in the patient's blood. Several different sorts are found and three are highly significant for lupus.

  1 *Antiphospholipid antibody syndrome* (APS – a syndrome is a group of symptoms that occur together). Another name for this is 'sticky' blood syndrome or Hughes' syndrome after Graham Hughes, head of the Lupus Research Clinic at St Thomas' Hospital in London, and one of the foremost experts on the disease (see his books in 'Further reading'). In 1983 Dr Hughes' team described a disorder characterized by blood clotting in both arteries and veins. Pregnant patients with the problem had a tendency to recurrent miscarriage and everyone was at higher risk of stroke (when a clot of blood that has formed in a blood vessel breaks loose and travels to the brain, causing loss of function and sometimes death). APS affects perhaps 1 to 2 per cent of the general population, but a very high proportion of lupus patients, to the extent that its presence is highly suggestive, if not conclusive, of the disease. The discovery was also important because it showed that not all the features of lupus were caused by inflammation. (More about APS antibodies in Chapter 10.)

  2 About 40 to 50 per cent of patients have an antibody known as anti-Sm (the 'Sm' has no medical meaning; it comes from the name of the patient in whom it was first identified). Again this test is not particularly sensitive (a high percentage of

people with the disease do not test positively) but it may again be unique to lupus, hence highly specific (no false positives).

3 Elevated levels of anti-DNA, an antibody to the basic building block of life (deoxyribonucleic acid, found in the nucleus of all human cells), occur in at least 50 per cent of people with lupus at some stage. Some researchers believe it may be unique to lupus, making it highly specific, though not particularly sensitive (many lupus sufferers test negatively).

4 Finally, there is an antibody found at high levels in the blood of people with lupus that, although not exclusive to them, is considered so significant that it warrants the status of an ACR diagnostic criterion. *Antinuclear antibodies (ANA)* appear to react indiscriminately against material released from the nucleus of a cell when it has been destroyed. Although patients with other diseases – rheumatoid arthritis, liver disease and some infections, as well as those on some drugs – also react positively to this test, a very high proportion of lupus patients (in some studies between 90 and 100 per cent) test positive, which makes it one of the most sensitive tests available, although again, not highly specific. Yet another sign that an abnormal degree of cell destruction has taken place (all that broken furniture) is the presence of unusually high levels of freely circulating DNA in the blood of lupus patients. DNA properly belongs *inside* the nucleus of a whole cell, not wandering about in the bloodstream.

The antibodies detected in the last two tests are noteworthy and distinctive. They are not the kind present in the blood because the patient had been exposed to and fought off an infection like TB. Nor are they the kind stimulated deliberately by vaccination to protect people against a future attack of an illness like measles. These are antibodies characteristic of autoimmune conditions; antibodies that do battle with the body's own cells. These antibodies don't react to intact tissues and organs, but to broken-down pieces of cells released during the autoreactive battle.

With few exceptions normal cells in the body die eventually; the body is in a continual process of renewing and replacing itself, disposing of old, worn-out cells and budding-out new ones, all with no disruption to the smooth running of the body as a whole. The process of normal, programmed cell death is known as *apoptosis*, from two Greek words that mean 'falling away'. One avenue that scientists are exploring is that in autoimmune diseases something goes wrong with normal apoptosis. Instead of quietly falling away, 'elderly' cells totter on in a decrepit state, and these continue to promote inflammation and abnormal autoreactive activity (see Chapter 11).

Other signs, other diagnostic techniques

The author regrets that this has been a long, rather difficult chapter and that it isn't over yet. Spare a minute for this bit, even if you have skipped a few of the complicated antibody tests that have gone before.

Some symptoms that aid diagnosis used to be on the ACR list but have been dropped. One is hair loss. About a quarter of lupus patients experience this though there can be alternative explanations. Another is a condition known as *Raynaud's phenomenon*, which is a bit like frostbite and can exist independently as well as in association with lupus. Raynaud's phenomenon is caused by a spasm of small blood vessels – *vasospasm* – which shuts off the circulation to the extremities, usually the fingers, occasionally ears, nose or toes, so that they turn white, then blue with cold, and red and painful. There is more about this condition in Chapter 9.

Other significant changes may show up in the blood of lupus patients; for example, the amount of complement – the antibody support-troops who figured in the description of inflammation earlier in this chapter – may be depleted as a result of prolonged inflammation, and there are other more interesting, though not specific, antibodies that may add support to a diagnosis. But for now that's quite enough antibodies.

The St Thomas' criteria

Before you can move on from diagnosis to the important business of how lupus patients are treated, we would like to return for a moment to the 'eye of the experienced beholder worth a laboratory-load of tests' that we met in the box 'Diagnosis – craft or science', in Chapter 4 (see p. 32). Graham Hughes – who heads the lupus unit at St Thomas' Hospital and who was responsible for identifying

Hughes' syndrome – says that the ACR list, although invaluable for the purpose of *classifying* lupus, is restrictive when it comes to diagnosis. 'It narrows the scope for lateral thinking in clinical medicine, something which lupus, above all, allows us in abundance', he says. Dr Hughes has drawn up an alternative diagnostic list of 14 symptoms (11 listed below) that may be detected in the surgery from observation or the patient's history. They have, he admits, no statistical justification. They are based 'solely on the experiences gained in a huge clinical practice'. (He also lists additional evidence that may be noted in laboratory tests. These are not included.)

- **'Growing pains'.** In the UK this is a label widely used for joint pains in teenage life. While usually considered benign, it is often sufficiently severe for the child to be taken to the doctor. Some patients give a history of 'rheumatic fever' – a label that persists in the UK despite the condition's almost total disappearance.
- **Teenage migraine.** This symptom is associated with the antiphospholipid (Hughes') syndrome. Many patients over 30 with cerebro-vascular accidents (blood clots flying to the brain) give a past history of recurrent abortions in their twenties and 'migraine' in their teens.
- **'Glandular fever'.** Prolonged periods off school due to so called 'glandular fever' is a recurrent theme.
- **Severe reaction to insect bites.** 'The skin is a major organ affected by lupus. It would be surprising if hypersensitivity to insect bites were not an important phenomenon in lupus', says Dr Hughes.
- **Recurrent miscarriages.** 'To be precise, this criterion is not truly a lupus criterion, but is an indicator of those lupus patients with the antiphospholipid or Hughes' Syndrome. Indeed, in our lupus pregnancy clinic we believe that if APS patients are excluded, then lupus itself is not a cause of recurrent spontaneous abortion', admits Dr Hughes.
- **Septrin** (a common antibiotic drug) **or sulphonamide** (an old sulphur antibacterial drug) **allergy.** It is quite common for patients to report not only a history of severe rashes and other adverse reactions to septrin, but that the clinical onset of the disease coincided with their taking of the drug.
- **Agoraphobia** (fear of open spaces) or **claustrophobia** (fear of being in enclosed spaces). It is known that the central nervous

system is involved in lupus. Dr Hughes believes that evidence of abnormal fears in a patient's history indicate a pre-lupus warning. 'The history, varying from panic attacks in shops to fear of motorway driving, for example, is sometimes protracted, lasting months or years. In many cases, the history is not volunteered, or the episodes are considered unrelated or "something from the past" ', he says.

- **Finger flexor tendonitis** (difficulty in extending the fingers flat caused by joint and tendon inflammation). The patient says, 'I cannot say my prayers'. Dr Hughes values it as a lupus pointer because it varies from the pattern of finger-joint inflammation seen in other connective-tissue diseases like rheumatoid arthritis.
- **Premenstrual exacerbations** (problems). All rheumatic diseases are influenced by the menstrual cycle, and none more so than lupus. Some patients are almost immobilized during the two to three days preceding menstruation. Dr Hughes says, 'It is my practice in some cases to alter the dose of medication during this time. Although difficult to quantify, I believe that significant premenstrual disease flare is sufficiently prominent in lupus to be included in this alternative list.'
- **Family history of autoimmune disease.** This is self-evident common sense. Dr Hughes comments: 'In old-fashioned history-taking, the family history is important. Lupus is genetically determined, and the presence of other autoimmune diseases in the family (including thyroid disease) is worthy of inclusion in the clinical scoring system.'
- **Dry Shirmer's test** (the doctor sticks a sliver of blotting paper into the lower eyelid). 'It is highly irritant and only if the patient has some abnormality of the tear duct – as in lupus or *Sjögren's syndrome* – will the paper remain dry. In a patient with vague or non-specific symptoms, a bone-dry Shirmer's test points towards one of the autoimmune diseases.'

Dr Hughes' three remaining criteria relate to highly significant laboratory tests. In conclusion, Dr Hughes says: 'All of us can diagnose lupus in the presence of a butterfly rash, *nephritis* (kidney disease) and alopecia (hair loss). The challenge comes at the other end of the spectrum; the atypical case; the mild case; the differential between real disease versus no organic disease whatsoever; the ailing teenage daughter of a known lupus patient.'

6

Treating lupus with drugs 1
– keeping the wolf from the door

Lupus is a fiendish beast to track down, hence the immense effort to
arrive at a diagnosis. Once the doctors are pretty sure they have it in
their sights, however, the plan of attack can be made. Lupus has
many manifestations and treatment is inevitably tailored to the
severity of the patient's symptoms, but the pharmacy from which aid
is drawn comprises four main drug groups:

- painkilling non-steroidal anti-inflammatory drugs (NSAIDs)
- antimalarials
- steroids
- immunosuppressants.

Up to the middle of the last century, lupus was so poorly understood
that doctors had little science to guide them and adopted the 'let's-
see-if-this-will-do-any-good' principle not unknown today. Serendipity and the law of averages mean that such pragmatism quite
often produces a hit. There may also be disasters, and success via
serendipity does not advance our understanding of the disease
process greatly. The other snag of the approach is that even when a
drug appears to work against some symptom of a disease,
unanticipated, harmful side effects, or the emergence of subgroups
of people who are particularly vulnerable to them, only emerge later.
These are some of the reasons why these days *therapeutics* – that is,
treatment of illness with drugs – advances by means of properly
controlled trials which demonstrate effectiveness and side effects
before new, experimental treatments are licensed for general use
(see box overleaf, 'Randomized clinical trials (RCT) – the therapeutic Gold Standard').

Problems of poly-pharmacy

Before looking at the drugs used to treat the various symptoms
associated with lupus, a word about taking drugs in general. Most of
us get used to taking a paracetamol for a headache, a course of

Randomized clinical trials (RCT) – the therapeutic Gold
Standard

The idea of using scientific method to test the effectiveness of drugs
or other medical procedures is a relatively modern concept. Witch
doctors apart, curing people has historically been as much about
faith and luck as medical understanding or effective treatment. But
as the causes and mechanisms of disease emerged from mystery
and superstition, so the physician's ability to alter the course of
disease predictably increased: to intervene – to use a favourite
medical word.

The first example of what is now regarded as the Gold Standard
for clinical trials – the randomized, controlled trial, or to give it its
high-carat denomination, *the randomized, placebo-controlled, double-blind, trial* – took place just after the Second World War in 1948
when Austin Bradford Hill set up a trial of streptomycin, an antibiotic
derived from soil fungi discovered a few years previously, to
measure its effectiveness in TB. Patients with advanced pulmonary
(lung) TB were randomly assigned to one of two treatment groups. If
doctors are allowed to choose which patients receive a new active
drug and which are allocated to the control group on standard
treatment, there is always the risk they will put the patients with the
best prognosis into the active group, thus skewing the outcome.
When, in addition to patients being randomly assigned to either
treated or control group, they don't know whether they are on the
active drug or not, the trial is known as 'blind'. If, in addition, the
medical team looking after the patient and running the study is not
told which patient is in which group, the study is 'double-blind';
neither the patient nor the medical staff know who is in which group.
This prevents any hidden psychological bias for or against the

antibiotics for cystitis, or an antihistamine because we get hay fever,
but these common medications are all taken in response to
recognized symptoms, taken alone, and stopped once the symptoms
subside – or once the course is complete in the case of antibiotics.
The drugs prescribed for lupus are less symptom-specific. In
addition, lupus patients have the same common ailments requiring
medication as the rest of the population so at times they may find
themselves with a veritable chemist shop laid out on the dressing

new treatment. Clinical studies usually measure the effect of a new treatment against a *comparator*: either the standard treatment of the day – it would not be ethical to withhold all treatment from a sick person for research purposes – or, in non-fatal conditions, unlike TB, against a non-active dummy pill (a *placebo*) to conceal from them whether they are taking the active treatments or not. Patients with some illnesses – depression, for example – may show marked improvement when receiving a placebo. This response to treatment, albeit with a non-active compound, is called the *placebo effect*.

In the Hill study of streptomycin, 107 patients were enrolled. When the results were un-blinded it was discovered that 14 of the 52 patients on standard treatment had died (these were very ill people remember) but that only 4 of the 55 patients who had been given the active drug had died. Streptomycin really worked.

The supremacy of the RCT was reinforced in the early 1950s by trials of the Salk polio vaccine tested using an elaborate double-blind trial on nearly 2 million US children. These early successes, together with early failures of clinical testing procedures – thalido-mide, an effective drug for morning sickness in early pregnancy, was found to have damaged the foetus developing in the womb – led to standards for testing experimental drugs being enshrined in European and United States law. These days, before a drug is approved for general use it must be tested against these standards. 'Randomized, placebo-controlled, double-blind trials are the appro-priate means, indeed almost the only scientific means, to establish the efficacy of a treatment' (David Healy, *The Antidepressant Era*, Harvard University Press, 1997).

table. What's more, the fatigue and emotional ups and downs that often accompany lupus play havoc with memory and attention. The advice of the experts is: 'Write your medication schedule down: which pill, how many and at which time of day; whether before or after food. Write them all down and, ideally, tick them off as they go down.' You should probably also make a note of any drug that doesn't agree with you. Some drugs can increase photosensitivity for example, already a problem for many with lupus; others produce side effects like stomach upsets or rashes in *some* people. If you are one, make sure you record the danger drugs and that they appear on your medical and dental notes.

The problem of poly-pharmacy (taking several drugs together or in regular succession) is not unique to people with lupus. The preventive regimens designed to protect against heart disease and other conditions of old age – the menopause, high blood pressure, raised cholesterol, diabetes, for example – mean that many of us stand before the serried ranks of pills in middle age. Lupus patients are old lags at it long before that.

Charlotte's story
In the long hot summer of 1976 Charlotte was outdoors revising for her A-levels. She developed a fiery rash and felt generally unwell, but somehow she managed to keep going and only went to the doctor once the holidays had started. At once he recognized the classic butterfly rash, organized a battery of tests and told Charlotte she had lupus. The symptoms subsided during the holidays with little medication. Charlotte went off for her 'gap' year, back-packing across Europe. Somewhere in what was then Yugoslavia she developed cystitis and found herself trying to communicate with a local doctor in the rudimentary German they both spoke. 'Keine penicillin', insisted Charlotte, who knew she was allergic to the drug. Unfortunately she couldn't remember the name of the antibiotic that her family doctor did prescribe for her. She certainly didn't know the German for lupus. The local doctor prescribed a sulphonamide antibiotic and within two days Charlotte broke out in a rash; not just her face, but her hands, lower arms and her ankles. It was November and the sun was low, but the drug had potentiated Charlotte's photosensitivity.

Non-steroidal anti-inflammatory drugs (NSAIDs)

The acronym NSAIDs – pronounced 'en-sayeds' – is used freely in talking about dear old aspirin and its younger brothers. They are used to treat such a wide range of conditions that two important things about them embodied in their cumbersome name are easily overlooked: they kill pain; they *also* reduce inflammation and do it without belonging to the *corticosteroid* family of drugs. Corticosteroids are also powerfully anti-inflammatory and very effective in the treatment of lupus (see Chapter 7). However, they pack a payload of side effects and they also have some rather disreputable relations: the anabolic steroids used by athletes to enhance performance.

In the first half of the twentieth century high doses of aspirin – the oldest member of the NSAID family – were the standard treatment for rheumatoid arthritis, juvenile arthritis and lupus patients with arthritic symptoms. However, once the dosage and side effects of these drugs were studied in properly controlled trials it emerged that good old aspirin had quite a few serious side effects. It irritates the lining of the gut causing indigestion and intestinal bleeding, and may also affect the liver. People with lupus, it appears, are more likely than most people to be prone to abnormal liver reactions to aspirin, especially in high doses, so the development of NSAIDs about forty years ago was welcomed by rheumatologists and arthritis sufferers alike.

NSAIDs suppress pain by interrupting the messages sent from the site of the pain to the brain. The cytokines – the chemical messengers that become so overexcited in rheumatic conditions – produce substances called *prostaglandins* that cause inflammation. Aspirin and the NSAIDs work by interrupting this process. That's why you will sometimes hear them called 'prostaglandin-inhibitors'. When production of prostaglandins is reduced, so is pain, swelling and stiffness. They are good as a first-line treatment for these symptoms because they are fast-acting. And as anyone who is a fan of aspirin knows, it offers pain relief within half an hour. Inflammation and swelling take a little longer, but they start to go down within a matter of a week or so.

Just as experienced users learn that one painkiller works better for them than another, even so trial and error are usually required to find which NSAID is effective and produces the least side effects for individual lupus patients, because NSAIDs also have side effects. The most common is indigestion, a result of the irritation the drug causes to the lining of the stomach which can ultimately lead to ulcers. More refined versions that aim to reduce inflammation without damaging the gastric lining have recently been developed and are known as 'coxibs'. (To learn how these work and about their drawbacks read the box 'Good and bad COX' overleaf.)

When NSAIDs are used to treat rheumatoid arthritis or lupus they are primarily being prescribed to reduce inflammation and are

49

required in higher doses than for a headache or muscle strain. Finding the right drug and establishing the effective dose with minimum side effects may take some time. Although these are for the most part tried and tested, common-or-garden drugs, some even obtainable without prescription over the counter at a chemist, in the doses used to treat arthritic symptoms they need close monitoring. In addition to the risk of a wide range of side effects, some people are allergic to them and they also interact with other drugs patients may be taking, so always report anything untoward to your doctor straight away.

It is estimated that as many as 30 million people worldwide take NSAIDs every day to control their pain and inflammation. Family doctors are familiar with their side effects.

Good and bad COX

NSAIDs work by blocking an enzyme known as *cyclo-oxygenase* (COX) which contributes to the production of prostaglandins which in turn release platelets that promote blood-clotting and protect the gut, kidneys and blood. This is why prostaglandin-inhibiting drugs can damage the gut and kidneys, producing the common side effects of increased gut-bleeding and upset stomach. A little more than twelve years ago, scientists discovered that there were in fact two sorts of COX enzyme: COX-1, which acts to protect the gastric lining, and COX-2, which is only found in inflamed tissue and which is produced in response to stimulation by those overexcited cytokines that characterize autoimmune diseases. The race was on to inhibit COX-2 – the bad guys – while leaving COX-1 to carry on the good work.

There are currently four COX-2 inhibitors (Coxibs) on the market (see box 'NSAIDs used to treat lupus' opposite) and two more are in the pipeline. To begin with there was much excitement about these improved NSAIDs; in clinical trials of people with arthritis they controlled pain and inflammation without as many nasty gastric side effects. However, in September 2004, follow-up research in a large number of patients revealed that there was a slightly increased risk of 'cardiovascular events' (that's heart attack or stroke) for those on one Coxib called rofecoxib or Vioxx, and the makers withdrew it.

NSAIDs used to treat lupus

First spare a thought for drug names. Drug names belong to no spoken language and are almost impossible for the lay person to pronounce or remember. They are assembled piecemeal by the people who develop them and are intended to provide clues as to what's in them or how they work. But they only do this for experienced pharmacologists. Just to complicate matters, each drug has at least two names: its chemical name – this is the name that describes its active ingredients – and its trade name, which, being a personal thing, takes an initial capital letter. Trade names are meant to be catchy and easier to pronounce than chemical names, but they often aren't. And they vary from country to country, which makes them even more difficult to recognize. There is an unspoken belief among doctors that patients don't really need to know more about their drugs than is included in the Patient Information Leaflet enclosed in the pack – with the apt acronym PIL. They think it will make you worry. But if you know the names of your drug and can get on the Internet you can find out a lot, both good and bad, about your medication.

NSAIDs: salicylates (aspirin – acetylsalicylic acid in fancy dress) (Aspro Clear, Bufferin, Ecotrin, Encaprin), ibuprofen, fenoprofen (Naflon), ketoprofen (Oruvail), piroxicam (Feldene), naproxen (Naprosyn), diclofenac (Voltarol), nabumetone (Relifex)

COX-2 inhibitors: celecoxib (Celebrex), valdecoxib (Bextra), etoricoxib (Arcoxia).
Rofecoxib (Vioxx) is the drug that has been withdrawn following the side-effect scare.
Lumiracoxib (Prexige) is currently still undergoing clinical trials.

Inevitably this raised question marks against the others. The argument goes that normally, although COX-1 tends to promote thrombosis (blood-clotting), it is inhibited by the action of COX-2, so that blocking COX-2 would suggest that unopposed COX-1 would indeed increase cardiovascular risk. On the other hand, inflammation is also implicated in cardiovascular events, and by that score controlling inflammation by blocking COX-2 should be protective. As usual with this sort of medical conundrum, 'further studies are called for'. Meanwhile, wise old GPs observe that not only are Coxibs now tarnished with the 'cardiovascular event' brush but that in practice some patients taking them still experience the gastric side effects they were supposed to avoid *and* they cost a great deal more than aspirin or standard NSAIDS. 'I foresee them disappearing from the scene', said one experienced doctor.

But pain is only the half of treating lupus – and NSAIDs only a quarter of the drug groups doctors prescribe. For more about more powerful drugs, turn to Chapter 7.

7

Treating lupus with drugs 2
– call the huntsman

Doctors are instinctively conservative. If they believe it is safe to 'wait and see', to avoid intervention and to allow the body to correct itself without medical assistance, they probably will. If the patient's symptoms – even temporary symptoms – are sufficiently severe to make 'wait and see' too miserable to endure, they will still choose the mildest of treatments first; the one with the least side effects. Only if matters become serious do they go in with the big guns. This is why we have discussed NSAIDs first for the treatment of lupus. Although not side-effect free, they are well known and comparatively mild. The other drugs in the lupus pharmacy have more serious potential side effects, but balancing this risk, they are generally more effective.

Antimalarial drugs are anti-lupus

The first group of drugs found to be helpful in lupus was originally designed to attack the malaria parasite: a great example of the serendipity that occasionally blesses the let's-see-if-this-will-have-any-effect-on-it approach to therapeutics. The oldest antimalarial – quinine – was tried experimentally in lupus as early as the 1890s (see the box in Chapter 2, 'Lupus in history'), and related drugs were used successfully to heal the skin lesions associated with discoid lupus in the 1920s. Several quinine derivatives are still prescribed today, particularly hydroxychloroquine (Plaquenil), chloroquine (Nivaquine, Aralen) and mepacrine (Atabrine). Of the three, hydroxychloroquine is most commonly prescribed because it has the lowest side-effect profile.

Treating malaria in its active phase involves bringing down fever, so perhaps it is not surprising that antimalarials do this for lupus sufferers too. But they also help the skin lesions, joint inflammation and fatigue. Characteristically for a serendipitous discovery, there is no clear explanation as to why they should have this effect. They are immunosuppressive. (A study done in Africa showed that antimalarials used conventionally to treat active malaria damp down the response to vaccination – when a protective immune response is the desired effect.) They are also antiviral and anti-inflammatory, though via what mechanism is unclear; possibly by damping down the production of prostaglandins (as do NSAIDs) or those chemical messengers of inflammation, the cytokines (see Chapter 5). They have two other clearly beneficial actions: they are sun-blocking – valuable to lupus sufferers who are so often hypersensitive to light – and they lower cholesterol, one of the soluble fats transported in the bloodstream which contribute to cardiovascular disease and the production of blood clots. This is good news for people with lupus who often have clotting problems, especially during pregnancy, and good news for everyone else too.

... and the bad news

There are of course side effects. In the case of antimalarial drugs there is a small risk of the usual tummy upsets (about one patient in five), ringing in the ears (*tinnitus*) and occasionally headaches, but the major concern is damage to the retina of the eye.

When hydroxychloroquine is first prescribed it is usually given in quite high doses – up to 400 milligrams (mg) a day – and it can cause temporary visual problems: blurred vision or a 'halo effect' around lights. This is reversed once the dose is reduced. Finding the optimal dose for antimalarials is quite difficult because the drug does not become effective for at least two weeks, sometimes longer, so to begin with this starter side effect can be decisive. Graham Hughes employs a 'juggling' drug regimen with antimalarials if a patient has severe skin complications, and if 400 mg of hydroxychloroquine daily causes vision problems he reduces the dose by using a different antimalarial (mepacrine) on alternate days. (Mepacrine, also known as quinacrine, is not a first-choice antimalarial because it also has its own, different, vision side effects and can produce slight yellowing of the skin and eye-whites.)

The more serious vision side effect of antimalarials was seen more frequently in the past when high doses were used with less caution. It takes the form of pigment deposits in the retina – the area at the back of the eye where images are formed and relayed to the brain. This condition is called *macular retinopathy* and if allowed to continue undetected can lead to blindness. For this reason most hospitals keep a close check on patients on the drug. They are advised to protect their eyes from strong light *of all sorts* and *at all times*; to wear high-quality sunglasses, indoors as well as out, especially if they may be exposed to fluorescent or halogen lighting. In addition the eyes should be examined regularly by a qualified ophthalmologist. The frequency of such examinations could be as little as a few months, but not less than once a year.

If these precautions are observed there is evidence that antimalarials may be taken for months, or even years, and that in addition they may protect against lupus 'flares'.

Dougal's story
Dougal developed lupus in middle age. At first he put the arthritic symptoms down to wear and tear; it was only when the distinctive discoid rash appeared on Dougal's scalp that his doctor realized that it was lupus. Hydroxychloroquine was prescribed and after a few weeks the symptoms cleared up. But when the medication stopped the symptoms returned. Dougal went back onto the antimalarial, this time for months. It was only when he came to have his routine eye test nearly a year later that the ophthalmic optician discovered that there was damage to the retina. Dougal had noticed nothing untoward; as far as he was concerned his sight was normal. His doctor changed the medication, very apologetic that he had not insisted on Dougal having an ophthalmic check-up sooner. Subsequent eye-checks showed that the damage was not progressing. Dougal had been lucky; sometimes the sight continues to deteriorate even when the drug is stopped.

In the past antimalarials were always discontinued during pregnancy because of the risk that they might affect the developing foetus. However, an increasing number of studies now suggest that successful pregnancies can be completed by women taking hydroxychloroquine, though some obstetricians still prefer to err on the side of caution.

Corticosteroids

Does the hair stand up on the back of your neck at the mention of these drugs? Once highly thought of, they have acquired a bad reputation. When the first drug – *cortisone* – was launched in the

1940s it demonstrated such dramatic reductions in inflammation that it was hailed as a wonder drug, a 'cure' for rheumatoid arthritis and lupus, and earned its discoverers, Philip Hench and Edward Kendall, a Nobel Prize.

But in the wake of the rave reviews for the miracle cure came serious side effects – because the drugs were being used in very high doses at this time: weight-gain, raised blood pressure, easy bruising and slow healing, cataracts, muscular weakness, raised blood sugar causing problems with diabetes, less resistance to infection because the immune system was being damped down and, with long-term use, thinning of the bones – osteoporosis. Corticosteroids were no longer flavour of the month.

Corticosteroids are, in fact, chemical versions of hormones occurring naturally in the body. Human steroids are produced mostly by the adrenal glands, but also by the testicles and ovaries. They help control *metabolism* – how the body generates energy and disposes of waste – the development of sexual characteristics, immune function, the balance of fluids in the body and its tolerance of stress. There are many steroids with different functions: the sex hormones – testosterone, oestrogen and progesterone – adrenal cortical hormones, bile acids, sterols, anabolic agents and oral contraceptives are all steroids. Corticosteroids are not the same as anabolic steroids, the ones taken by weightlifters to build muscle. The role of corticosteroids is protective: they maintain the fluid balance in the body and help it cope with stress; along the way they reduce inflammation.

Doses and delivery regimen

In the treatment of lupus, the role of steroids is anti-inflammatory. Nowadays the pros and cons of corticosteroids are better understood and their use, delivery and dosage have been refined. They have probably advanced the treatment of lupus more than any other drug, and almost every person with lupus will take them at some time or other, on a short- or a long-term basis. Doctors prescribing them follow strict guidelines.

Getting the dose right – not too much, not too little – is central to the administration of steroids. Inflammation is the healthy response to infection, so that if it is suppressed (by drugs) the patient becomes vulnerable to infection; hence it is essential that the dose is kept as low as is effective. In Graham Hughes' experience, a seriously ill patient may briefly require as much as 60 mg daily, reducing to 40–30 mg after one or two weeks. Milder cases might receive 15–20 mg daily for the first few weeks, reducing to a maintenance dose of 5–10 mg a day. Reducing the daily dose of steroids must always be done gradually and with the co-operation of the patient. It is possible to reduce high doses on a steeper gradient, but a below 20 mg reduction must always be extremely gradual – by as little as 1 mg a month – in Graham Hughes' practice. (This fine-tuning can be hampered by the difficulty of sourcing 1 mg tablets, requiring the patient's co-operation in executing neat pill sections with a razor blade.)

A number of steroid drug regimens may be employed. They are most commonly taken by mouth and the most widely used drug is prednisolone (or prednisone). ACTH (adreno-cortico-trophic-hormone) is an injectable form of steroid which is administered twice weekly, and methylprednisolone is given via a drip into a vein. This can obviously only be done in hospital, but for seriously ill people can be a useful way of delivering large doses of steroids with surprisingly few side effects. (When steroids are taken by mouth they are available in a coated form to reduce the usual unpleasant gastric side effects.) At the other end of the dose scale is the practice of prescribing steroids to be taken on alternate days, to allow the natural source of steroids – the person's own adrenal glands – to re-boot. One of the principle side effects of steroid treatment is that the body, recognizing that large amounts of the stuff are washing around, cuts back on home production. This is why coming off steroids has to be done gradually; to let the adrenal glands limber up and get back into production.

Taking low-dose steroids, say 7.5 mg a day even for a limited period, causes other side effects. Two are quite common: sleep disturbance and increased appetite. As has been explained, steroids control metabolism – which in turn determines when energy and attention levels go up and when they come down – and, through this, the cycles of attention and sleepiness that constitute your body clock. Some people taking steroids find their body clocks totally reversed: wide awake at three in the morning and sleepy at three in the afternoon, as though they had been working the night shift or had just returned from the other side of the globe with jet lag.

Taking high doses of steroids over long periods cues the side effects that gave the drugs their bad name: muscle weakness, raised blood-sugar levels (sometimes full-blown diabetes) and osteoporosis. High doses are usually only given for acute emergencies in lupus, and rarely for more than a short period. (Treatment for osteoporosis is covered later.) One of the lesser-known side effects is mood disturbance: depression or the opposite – mania. If the family has a history of psychiatric problems it should always be reported to the physician before someone takes steroids.

Corticosteroid drugs used to treat lupus

Prednisone, prednisolone, methylprednisolone (Medrol), dexamethasone, triamcinolone, betamethasone, cortisone, hydrocortisone, and adreno-cortico-trophic-hormone (ACTH) injections.

Immunosuppressive drugs

Lupus is an autoimmune disease, so you might think it obvious that it should be treated with immunosuppressive drugs. In fact immunosuppressants were developed for a quite different medical condition. Fifty years ago, when the first successful human organ transplants took place, rejection was a great problem. The body receiving the transplant recognized the organ as a foreigner and the immune system attacked it. Drugs to suppress this natural process were essential if transplanted organs were to survive. Some drugs already in existence were found to have immunosuppressant action (serendipity scores again) and others have been developed since. These have been tried as treatment for other conditions like rheumatoid arthritis and lupus where an overactive immune system is part of the problem. In lupus they clamp down on the over-production of B-cells producing antibodies. They also interfere with rapidly dividing, proliferating (multiplying) cells, hence are also used to treat cancer.

Immunosuppressants are used in much lower doses to treat autoimmune diseases than for organ transplant rejection or cancer. Nevertheless these are potent drugs and their powerful action may spread to other healthy cells which are not their designated target.

Their side effects are considerable, so they are only given if the disease becomes serious; if the kidneys become inflamed (*nephritis*), for example, or if milder drugs are ineffective, and always under very close medical supervision and with constant monitoring.

The two immunosuppressants used most frequently to treat lupus are azathioprine (Imuran) and cyclophosphamide (Endoxana, Cytoxan). Two others may be used as backup – methotrexate (Folex, Mexate, Rheumatrex) and cyclosporin (Neoral, Sandimmune). A third, relatively new drug – mycophenolate mofetil, or MMF (CellCept) – has distinguished itself in the support of kidney transplants and looks promising in the treatment of lupus, although it has yet to establish a long track record.

Azathioprine

This is the immunosuppressant used most widely in the management of lupus. Although it lowers resistance to infection, it has an otherwise quite acceptable side-effect profile and has even been used for children with lupus and sometimes for pregnant women. The dose given is related to body-weight: usually between 100 and 150 mg a day. It has been used to treat nephritis and has been continued successfully for a period of years. On the evidence of blood tests it also appears to have a beneficial effect on other aspects of lupus.

Cyclophosphamide

Studies over the past twenty years suggest that this drug is even more effective than azathioprine, especially when it comes to life-threatening kidney disease, and it is the most likely to be prescribed when heavy-duty therapy is indicated. It may be taken by mouth, like azathioprine, or by injection, often by what is known as *pulse therapy*. This involves delivering relatively high doses of the drug straight into the vein (intravenously) at specific intervals: of days, weeks or months. It may also be used in conjunction with another drug: an antimalarial, or a corticosteroid like prednisolone or methylprednisolone. This last combination has been very successful in maintaining prolonged lupus remissions.

Methotrexate and *Cyclosporin*

Methotrexate has revolutionized the treatment of rheumatoid arthritis because of its powerful affect upon joint inflammation. It can be helpful in lupus if arthritis is the chief problem and may also help with skin rashes, but is not the drug of first choice for the condition. Cyclosporin, which modifies the immune system in a slightly different way from other immunosuppressants, may be helpful in some cases of lupus, but on the downside it carries serious and distinctive side effects, one of which is raised blood pressure. Since this is a major problem in lupus patients with kidney involvement, cyclosporin is definitely at the bottom of the list for lupus.

Mycophenolate mofetil or MMF (CellCept)

By contrast, this addition to the immunosuppressant drug list has recently moved sharply up in favour. Launched initially, like its brothers, to treat organ rejection after transplant, the first studies to demonstrate its use in the treatment of autoimmune disease were published in 2003. It showed itself to be as effective, if not more so, than pulse therapy cyclophosphamide and with a much lower side-effect profile.

For obvious reasons new drugs are first used on the most seriously ill patients, often those who have failed to respond to standard drug therapy, on the principle of 'nothing to lose'. MMF was compared with cyclophosphamide for the treatment of lupus patients with severe kidney disease. The newer drug's reduced side effects gave it another leg-up over the older drug: fewer patients withdrew from treatment. All too often distressing side effects contribute to patients deciding that they would rather come off the drug than put up with them any more; what doctors call *non-compliance*. The most effective drug is useless if patients can't stand taking it.

It remains to be seen if MMF will prove as successful in treating patients with less severe manifestations of lupus: patients with less to lose by abandoning treatment.

Treating drug side effects

Of course, people with lupus don't have to give up a drug to avoid side effects. Some can be treated with yet more drugs.

Infection

Immunosuppressants and corticosteroids reduce the body's ability to fight infection by depressing the production of white blood cells in the bone marrow. Every effort is made to avoid lupus patients on these drugs being exposed to infection. The herpesviruses which cause shingles and cold-sores are a particular problem but they can be treated with an anti-viral called acyclovir. Cystitis (inflammation of the bladder), another common problem with pulsed cyclophosphamide, responds to a drug called mesna. Bacterial infections can be treated with antibiotics.

High blood pressure

Nothing is more important for lupus patients with kidney involvement than controlling blood pressure. To do it justice, this requires a book to itself. Fortunately there are now very reliable, low side-effect treatments for it. The regime that suits lupus patients with kidney problems best is a *diuretic* a drug that reduces the amount of water retained in the tissues – plus a *calcium antagonist* which works on the walls of blood vessels to reduce pressure.

High blood cholesterol

Half the population of the UK has a blood cholesterol level that puts it at risk of coronary heart disease, so most of us are aware of the value of reducing the fat – particularly bad, saturated fats (the ones in dairy produce and meat) – in the diet. Elevated cholesterol is even more of a risk for lupus sufferers and fortunately there is a class of drug known as *statins* which support a healthy diet and may provide a range of other benefits as well. Needless to say, on no account should a person with lupus smoke. It is a major aggravation of high cholesterol, high blood pressure and heart disease.

Osteoporosis

This loss of bone density leading to easy fracturing and poor healing is one of the most serious results of prolonged or heavy use of steroids. Most patients on long-term steroid treatment have regular bone-density scans and take calcium (bone-building chemical) supplements and vitamin D supplements to help their body metabolize the calcium. If these are not sufficient a drug from a group called *bisphosphonates* – alendronate (Fosamax) or risadronate (Actonel) – may be prescribed.

People with lupus who also have antiphospholipid (Hughes') syndrome have a major problem with thrombosis (blood clots), and usually have to take medication to counteract this called *anticoagulants*. These are discussed in Chapter 10.

61

8
DIY lupus management – taming the wolf

This is a book about coping with a chronic illness. We've talked about research, doctors, laboratory tests and drugs. They are all there to inform and help you. But when you come home from the hospital or surgery and go through your front door, you are on your own. Day-to-day coping is up to you, supported by the friends and family we hope gather round you.

This chapter is in some ways the most important one in the book. Yes, you need to know what lupus is all about, but above all you need the strength and resourcefulness to grapple with the wolf in his lair, take him by the scruff, give him a good shake and then put a lead on him. He will always be with you, but you can make him walk to heel.

To begin with it will seem daunting. It may feel as though your life will never be the same again. Persevere. Break the problems down into bite-size pieces and deal with them one by one. Each person with lupus will have different priorities. For one the fatigue will be the major obstacle, for another the painful joints. Yet another may feel devastated by the damage to self-esteem caused by the skin rashes. Or maybe it is the moods that get you, the headaches, the gut upsets. Whatever your particular bug-bear there is something you, as well as the doctors and the drugs, can do to overcome it. Being active in disease management is empowering; it restores your self-confidence. It doesn't mean you can't ask for help if you need it. Getting constructive advice from experts, from family, friends or colleagues is a practical coping strategy in itself.

'I feel tired all the time!'

Fatigue is probably the most common symptom of lupus and the most intractable. How can you find the energy to cope when you feel like a wet dishcloth all the time? Take comfort in the fact that medication almost always helps. Once the drugs start to take effect, things begin to feel better. Get the doctors to check that you are not anaemic or have a lower-than-normal level of thyroid hormones or essential minerals, which can be corrected.

Meanwhile take stock of your life. Lupus fatigue is known by a variety of names: super-fatigue; wipe-out fatigue; a different kind of tired. Acknowledge it, and then treat it – with rest if necessary, in whatever dose is required. Note down the situations or activities that make you feel most exhausted, and find ways of avoiding them, modifying them or correcting the fatigue they cause.

Gillian's story

Gillian is a financial high-flier, a specialist in private/public partnerships. When lupus struck in her early thirties her biggest problem was business travel. It was bad enough commuting to and from London from her home in Cambridgeshire, but crossing time zones and then being expected to be bright and bushy-tailed in a business meeting immediately after was impossible. 'I got the company to let me do at least three days a week home-working', she explains. 'My laptop is networked so that I am in touch with everyone wherever I am, but I don't have to sit on the train for two hours every day to go into the office. Working from home is so much more flexible. If I need a nap, I can take it. If it's easier to work at night – the steroids sometimes do that to me – no one bothers; they pick up my messages when they come in the following morning. As for business trips to New York, or worse, to Tokyo, I allow an extra day so that I can sleep for at least ten hours before I have to perform. And of course, I tend to increase the drug dose before these testing times.'

Coping with fatigue, as Gillian found, is a mixture of cessation, adaptation and compensation. Don't drive yourself and don't blame yourself. If you have always been a busy, industrious person it is important to tell yourself that rest is therapy, not laziness, let alone sin. Lupus fatigue should not be ignored in some mistaken stoicism or guilt trip.

'I look so ghastly!'

An illness that affects the skin, especially the skin of the face, is devastating because, in addition to the discomfort, it dents your self-image. You don't just feel ill – often, you know you look ill.

Fortunately medication usually banishes a lupus rash, and there is a lot you can do yourself to make sure it stays that way. Once again it involves noting down what prompts a lupus flare *in your case*. The most likely cause is light of some sort. More than a third of people with lupus are photosensitive. As with sunburn, the fairer your skin, the more likely you are to be vulnerable. It doesn't mean you have to stay indoors, but when outside you should probably wear long sleeves, trousers and a broad-brimmed hat, and use a high-factor sun cream generously and repeatedly where your skin is exposed. Surveys reveal that nearly everyone fails to use sufficient sunscreen, and the places most likely to be neglected are the temples, the ears and the back and sides of the neck. (Women, or men who follow a tolerant profession, could do worse than cultivate long hair and a fringe.) And when you choose a sunscreen make sure it is non-allergenic. People with lupus are more prone than most to allergies. Watch out for sunscreens that contain para-aminobenzoic acid (PABA) or padimate; quite a few people react badly to it.

You will gradually get to know your own limits, but until you do, approach high-reflectivity locations with extreme caution: beaches, ski slopes, boats. Reflected light can make them as lethal in winter as in summer. If you are a light-sensitive lupus sufferer you may also need to be wary of some forms of artificial light. Unshielded, fluorescent bulbs emit significant amounts of ultraviolet light, as do halogen lamps. One woman with lupus found that her skin was affected by repeated exposure to the 'flash bulb' in the photocopier – a hitherto unsuspected occupational hazard.

Like Charlotte (see Chapter 6), you may find that your photosensitivity is aggravated by certain drugs or foods. A list of things to watch out for appears in the box opposite, 'Things known to increase photosensitivity'.

Allergy is another trigger for the skin symptoms of lupus and, as we have explained, people with lupus are more prone to allergic reactions than average. The fact that we can absorb things via the skin has been exploited by drug manufacturers to advantage. (If a drug can enter the system this way it avoids having to pass through the hostile environment of the stomach.) However, the preservatives, colorants, perfumes and other additives used in cosmetics, after-shaves, detergents and a range of common manufactured compounds that come in contact with the skin in the course of modern life may prompt an allergic reaction and, in a lupus sufferer, a flare. Nail polish contains the same sulphonamides that sparked Charlotte's lupus; a whole range of cosmetic substances, including permanent hair colourings, have been known to set off allergies – again, especially among people with lupus.

It doesn't mean that you must go naked and unadorned henceforth. Nothing would be more likely to make you feel miserable about your appearance. It does mean that you should adopt an attitude of extreme caution and constant vigilance about what goes on your skin. In the kitchen, rubber gloves are de rigueur – those delicate, reverse-handed gloves used by doctors don't make you clumsy – and when you go shopping for cosmetics look for the hypo-allergenic ranges.

Things known to increase photosensitivity

Some foods that derive from plants that contain chemicals called *psoralens* may aggravate photosensitivity. The most prominent are lemons, limes, celery, parsnips, parsley and figs. Even people without lupus have been known to suffer nasty skin reactions if they have spilt fruit juice on their skin on a sunny day.

Drugs that have this effect are many. Those people with lupus are most likely to come across are antibiotics (not just the old sulpha drugs, but tetracyclines too), an NSAID called piroxicam, a diuretic (water pill) called hydrochlorothiazide, some blood-pressure medication, antidepressants and anti-seizure medication. Photosensitivity is always mentioned among the side effects listed in the Patient Information Leaflet (PIL) of a prescription drug. For a detailed list go to <http://www.emedicine.com/derm/topic108.htm>

If you do have a flare of your lupus rash the accessibility of the skin as a route for medication works to your advantage. Steroid skin creams – 1 per cent hydrocortisone creams are available, prescription free – reduce the itchiness of both malar and discoid rashes, and the side effects common with oral corticosteroids are rare with topical products. Calamine lotion is also helpful for itching, as are warm baths with colloidal oatmeal or a bath-oil rub, and some people find glycerine soap less drying than the regular kind. Sicca syndrome, also known as Sjögren's syndrome (see Chapter 9) after the physician who first described it, contributes to overall skin dryness. Ask your doctor to recommend an unperfumed pharmaceutical moisturizer, as opposed to a cosmetic product, that you can use regularly all over your body.

If DIY remedies fail you, there are two new immunosuppressive topical treatments that your doctor can prescribe: tacrolimus (Protopic) and pimecrolimus (Elidel). These creams are not steroids and so far (they were only launched in 2002) appear to have minimal side effects.

'Sometimes I'm so depressed I want to die'

Being ill makes anyone feel fed up. The realization that you are not only ill and it hurts, and it's mucking up your life, but that it could well go on for the rest of your life, is like a prison sentence.

In fact people with lupus are not depressed solely as a reaction to having the illness. The disease itself can cause problems in the brain that lead to depression. People diagnosed with lupus often have a history of depression, and the good news is that it lifts once they are treated. The bad news is that some treatments – steroids, for example – can in themselves cause mood disruption. Disease and treatment don't affect everyone in the same way. If you do continue to feel disabling depression once your lupus is treated your doctors may suggest antidepressant drugs, at least while you come to terms with things.

However, you yourself can help your body cope with your feelings.

Exercise

One of the most effective ways of lifting mood is with exercise. Since exercise is also a helpful way to maximize movement and range in arthritic joints and an even better way to stave off the risk of osteoporosis, it comes highly recommended for people with lupus. Some people also find it helps with fatigue, and exercise is, of course, to be recommended for everyone who values a healthy lifestyle.

It's a well-known fact that exercise gives you a natural high. Some people become addicted to it, exercise to achieve it, and feel down if they can't get their regular fix of it. The explanation is thought to be that exercise releases natural body chemicals called *endorphins*. These appear to reduce pain and generally to lift the spirits. Exercise also concentrates the mind because it involves effort. Unpleasant, intrusive thoughts recede. Your mind and body become focused on the present. Those who don't exercise are sceptical. Get into your exercise routine and discover the truth.

Exercise doesn't necessarily mean weights or the gym, though use of moderate weights – in the region of $2\frac{1}{2}$ lbs or a kilogram – can be helpful in warding off osteoporosis. Brisk walking, swimming, dancing and golf all keep the joints and muscles active, encourage deep breathing and occupy your mind pleasantly. If your joints are swollen you will need to strike a balance with rest and gentle exercise. If in doubt consult your doctor or a physiotherapist.

Don't cut yourself off from others

Which 'others' only you know. Keep doing things with the children; keep going to church or the football; keep singing with the choir and having your parents to lunch. Keep walking your dog or feeding the wild birds. Animals don't notice if you look funny or are not as lively as you were, and those who know you make allowances. Being with others encourages you to focus on other people and activities; something other than your own disrupted life. Doing things you enjoy or are good at establishes a continuity that counteracts those feelings of disruption and loss. When you switch the spotlight away from yourself, help someone else or solve a shared problem, you stop being a victim and become an actor in life again. And being an actor restores your self-esteem.

You could decide to join a lupus support group and by sharing your problems help yourself and maybe others. The West Midlands in the UK is particularly well supplied in this department, but organizations and websites listed under 'Useful addresses' at the end of the book will find help somewhere near you.

Give yourself rewards

Make a list of things you enjoy. It's difficult when you are low, and to start with you may have to enlist help. 'Remember how much you laughed at *Some Like It Hot*?' says your partner. Go out and get the video. Laughter is therapeutic. Write down favourite foods, favourite places, favourite things: stroking the cat, scented candles, long, hot baths. Find easy, little rewards to reach out for which will lift your spirits when you are down. Listing them is a valuable exercise in itself. It turns your attention towards positive, enjoyable experiences. With practice you can train yourself to *think* about good experiences as a way of driving out negative thoughts, especially if they keep you awake at night. If your imagination isn't up to conjuring up lying on the beach or listening to the nightingale, get yourself a soothing-sounds tape to send you to sleep.

Accentuate the positive

The principle behind *cognitive behaviour therapy* (*CBT*), one of the most successful forms of psychotherapy, is modifying how you think. Every situation can be interpreted in different ways. With practice you can turn negative thoughts back to front, as though you were arguing with someone. 'I so miss sunbathing' becomes 'I shall cultivate a pale and interesting look'. 'I'm such a burden on everyone' becomes 'I'm so lucky that everyone is so helpful'. To begin with you may need help, so start the argument with someone else, counsellor, partner or friend. Once you get the idea, every negative thought becomes a challenge: how can I turn it into a positive one?

'Choosing what to eat has become a minefield'

Both lupus and lupus medication can upset your stomach, and it is even more important to eat sensibly if you have a chronic disease than ordinarily. In addition, you may have to deal with allergies, or foods that appear to prompt a flare. Nevertheless, it is important not to put too much emphasis on the role of food in illness. The phrase 'You are what you eat' is a wild exaggeration and has many delusions to answer for. It is possible to make yourself less healthy by eating too much of the wrong things, or too little of the right, but with few exceptions – bacterial contamination, genuine allergies or intolerances – food is neither the cause of disease nor a cure for it.

Nevertheless, you will be bombarded by books, magazine articles and sites on the Internet that promise instant response from the introduction or removal of some dietary element, quite possibly costing you big money. Take it all with a very large pinch of salt. (Don't take too much real salt because that could be bad for fluid retention and your blood pressure.) Studies of large numbers of people with lupus are the most reliable source of information. But you will not necessarily conform to the norm. People can be very passionate about food, and if you believe that one food is making you feel better or another causing you flare-ups, it will do no harm to follow your instincts.

How many calories?

Being overweight is good for no one, and especially anyone with inflamed joints, but apart from this general health proviso there is little evidence that quantity of food affects lupus. There have been studies that suggested that fasting or a vegetarian diet might reduce arthritic symptoms but the studies were not very well controlled. There is sounder evidence when it comes to individual foods.

Fats

Graham Hughes reports the case history of a seriously ill rheumatoid arthritis patient who was passionate about cheese; she ate it every day. As a test, they tried withdrawing her daily cheese ration, in fact *all* dairy foods, for seven weeks. To everyone's surprise, within weeks there was a clinical improvement, so much so that in six months they were able to reduce her medication to zero. Being true scientists they decided that, to confirm the relationship between dairy produce and symptoms, they should give her cheese again – what is called 're-challenge' her symptoms. They tested her with several known food antigens with no response, finally giving her the cheese protein *casein*. Sure enough, the following day she was rigid with severe arthritis which lasted some days. She is now a healthy ex-cheese eater.

The effects of various sorts of fats in the diet have been studied in detail over the past decade. (In very crude terms, saturated=dairy =bad, and unsaturated=fish=good.) Fats are thought to affect the autoimmune system via their action on the prostaglandins which cause inflammation. A study in which people with lupus reduced their total fat intake to 25 per cent or less of their total daily food intake, which also included a fish-oil supplement, improved their symptoms over a three-month period. The explanation is thought to be that foods which have *antioxidant* and anti-inflammatory properties lessen arthritic symptoms. One of these, the latest star in the nutrition galaxy, is a fatty acid, omega-3, present in fish oils and some plant oils – walnut, almond, linseed and canola (rapeseed) – and has been shown to reduce the pain and swelling of autoimmune arthritis.

Vitamins

Fish oil is also rich in vitamin D, thought to have anti-inflammatory properties. Studies support the idea that vitamin D, which the body needs to absorb calcium, has a protective role in arthritis and also helps to reduce the osteoporosis caused by using corticosteroids. Bearing in mind that vitamin D is obtainable chiefly from sunlight, which lupus sufferers avoid, supplementing the vitamin via the diet makes a lot of sense. In addition to vitamin D, there is some evidence that a shortage of vitamin A may aggravate autoimmunity.

A lupus-drug diet

Diet is a very important way to counteract the effects of lupus medication. You have already been warned about steroids; the list of potential damage they can cause, especially taken in high doses and over long periods, makes very depressing reading, but even aspirin has a nutritional sting in its tail: it depletes vitamins A and B-complex. Diuretics and some NSAIDs can also do damage and all lupus medication carries a risk of upsetting digestion and damaging the lining of the gut. But let's be positive: you can compensate for these hazards with the right diet.

General rules

Take your drugs with food to decrease the irritating effect on the gut and to increase the time available for the absorption of the drug. Avoid excess fluid, limit saturated (dairy) fats, and eat plenty of fibre, fruit and vegetable to keep your weight down. Eat protein in moderation: meat sparingly, especially red meat, shellfish cautiously (oysters are a no-no for many lupus sufferers, and see scallops in 'Amber-light foods' opposite) but fish in quantity, especially when you have a fever which can cause nitrogen losses.

Green-light foods

To counteract the effect of lupus medication you need to boost potassium, calcium, zinc, iron and vitamins A, B-complex and B6, C, D and E. Fortunately these double up in a number of foods: fruit (especially bananas for potassium, oranges and strawberries for vitamin C), plums, blackberries, avocado and melon; vegetables, especially green ones: broccoli, spinach, cauliflower and green beans (with the exception of alfalfa sprouts, see p. 72); oily fish like salmon, herring, tuna and mackerel; high-fibre carbohydrates like wholegrain cereals, bread, nuts and potatoes.

Amber-light foods

Saturated fats – dairy produce and fatty meat – should appear in your diet in moderation or low-fat versions. Eggs, like meat and dairy foods, are high in cholesterol and should therefore keep a low profile; so are scallops, but they are too expensive and filling to eat in large quantities anyway.

Red-light foods

Salt (as little as is palatable): it increases fluid retention and can put up the blood pressure; mushrooms, cured meats and hot-dogs should be consumed with caution. They contain chemicals that have been found to aggravate lupus symptoms (also see oysters on the previous page).

Valerie, a lupus sufferer, was very positive about modifying her diet: 'I lost 11 kilos by reducing fat and increasing my intake of vitamins and potassium (fruits like bananas and oranges). I have fewer pains in the knees because of this weight loss, and the vitamins seem to reduce the butterfly rash on my face. Who knows if diet helps lupus, but if you carry too many kilos the pain is certainly more difficult to support. And now I feel better with other people too because I feel pretty in my new body. It's a morale booster.'

Are there no alternatives?

Wherever a chronic illness affecting many people is inadequately controlled by orthodox medicine you find the mushroom growth of alternative cures. It represents the capitalist marketing instinct responding to a natural human desire to try any port in a storm. Doctors are sceptical about such cures because they don't have to undergo the rigorous clinical testing demanded of a prescription medicine. The word 'natural' often used for such cures is little more than a word printed on the label. Many herbs and supplements – some Chinese medicines for example – contain potent ingredients (and ones that may interfere with prescribed and effective medication), but in unreliable quantities. Attempts to test the efficacy of such products are hampered by the fact that few have a consistent content from one batch to another. Investigations triggered by occasional cases of someone coming to serious harm after taking alternative products have revealed that they may contain substances, not mentioned in the labelling, such as powerful hormones, potent anti-inflammatories with major side effects, or sulpha drugs which set off hypersensitivity reactions and react with other drugs. Lupus expert Sheldon Blau quotes one supplement – alfalfa sprout – that, between the years 1995 and 2002, was associated with 17 outbreaks of food poisoning caused by *Salmonella* or *E-coli* infection that were reported to the Centers for Disease Control and Prevention in the USA. And of course people with lupus are particularly vulnerable because they are at more than average risk of suffering hypersensitive or allergic reactions to something like St John's wort, which can trigger severe photosensitivity.

Suffice to say that as a lupus sufferer you should be hyper-cautious about what you swallow – so-called alternative cures or food supplements – because you cannot be absolutely sure what's in them. If in doubt, don't take it.

Therapies that may help

Treat your digestive system with respect, but the outside of your body may indeed benefit from therapies not provided by orthodox medicine or physiotherapy. Relaxation and exercise techniques like yoga, t'ai chi, acupuncture, meditation or aromatherapy are undoubtedly stress-reducing and psychologically beneficial for a large number of chronic or incurable conditions, and acupuncture has demonstrated some painkilling effects. Many people with lupus, not to mention the unaffected, swear by them. A study of patients in North America and the UK, published in the journal *Arthritis & Rheumatism*, found that nearly half had tried alternative therapies. If you think you have found something that helps you and which doesn't clobber your bank account, it does no harm, provided you don't stop your prescribed medication.

9
Seven lupus-like conditions – sheep (and goats) in wolf's clothing

Lupus, as we have seen, is exceedingly difficult to pin down. It comes and goes, and in many guises. For years it was thought to be more than one disease, and even now the boundaries between lupus and lupus-like conditions are constantly shifting. The labelling of illnesses is an imperfect science, and is always under review.

The majority of people with lupus have lupus alone. Between 5 and 30 per cent of people with lupus have overlap symptoms. Connective tissue diseases (CTDs), which include lupus and rheumatoid arthritis, are particularly prone to this overlap phenomenon. Conditions like Raynaud's syndrome or Sjögren's may put in an appearance with lupus or a number of CTDs, and may also occur alone. What an individual patient is suffering from ultimately lands in the lap of the diagnosing physician. Fortunately treatment is driven by individual clinical symptoms, so does not vary greatly. Some of these conditions have already been mentioned and will be familiar.

CTDs have a number of features in common.

- They affect women much more frequently than men.
- They are 'multi-system': they affect the function of many organs.
- They overlap with one another, sharing symptoms, signs and abnormalities detected in the laboratory.
- Blood vessels are the most common target of injury.
- The abnormal behaviour of the immune system is responsible, at least in part, for the tissue damage caused.

Mixed Connective Tissue Disease (MCTD)

To the lay person this mouthful of a title probably seems a bit of an evasion. Graham Hughes calls it a 'mongrel' because it combines symptoms of lupus with those of other CTDs (see Chapter 1 and Chapter 4). It may include:

- Arthritis (especially of the hands – 'sausage fingers').
- Polymyositis-dermatomyositis PM-DM (muscle inflammation).
- *Scleroderma* (hardening of the skin or connective tissue).
- Raynaud's phenomenon (poor circulation leading to very cold extremities).

What distinguishes MCTD from lupus pure and simple is that it is almost never accompanied by the involvement of organs like the kidneys. Laboratory tests usually reveal that the patient has one specific antibody called 'antiRNP' but none of the other antibodies commonly associated with lupus, scleroderma or PM-DM. Although there is some doubt as to whether MCTD really is a separate disease or several diseases together in the same patient, the presence of the single antibody weights the scales in favour of a distinct disease.

MCTD treatment is geared to the symptoms experienced by each patient. But because the condition is less life-threatening than lupus or rheumatoid arthritis, doctors tend to be as conservative as possible in prescribing. Nevertheless, low to moderate doses of steroids are often required for many years to control MCTD adequately.

Raynaud's phenomenon – another of those conditions named after the doctor who first described it – may occur as part of MCTD, in conjunction with lupus (between 20 and 40 per cent of cases) or alone (between 5 and 10 per cent of the population). It's caused by the sudden constriction of the smallest arteries cutting off the peripheral circulation – an exaggerated version of the body's normal response to extreme cold and the need to conserve heat. In addition to practical measures – keeping the hands and feet well insulated in cold weather (some people use electrically heated gloves) – drugs that relax and dilate blood vessels can be helpful. Calcium antagonists, drugs originally designed to lower blood pressure and treat coronary heart disease, have been found particularly beneficial. Some doctors prefer to prescribe regular, low-dose aspirin as a preventative. This is also protective against coronary artery disease and stroke.

Sjögren's syndrome

Henrik Sjögren – nearest pronunciation: 'Shawgrun' – was a Swedish ophthalmologist and the first to recognize that people with CTDs often had dry eyes and mouth, or sicca (dry) syndrome (see

Chapter 4). The dryness is caused by a build-up of immune system cells in and around glands that produce tears and saliva leading to reduced production of these essential fluids. Some 5 per cent of lupus patients develop Sjögren's, sometimes late in life when most of their other symptoms have abated. The eyes feel gritty and itchy, especially early in the morning, and sometimes they are also sensitive to bright light. Some arthritis patients may also share one or more of the antibodies found in the blood of people with lupus. But discomfort is not the only symptom. Tears and saliva perform an important protective function and without them the eyes and teeth are more prone to infection. Saliva normally helps wash away plaque, the invisible bacterial film that develops on the surface of tooth enamel and leads to cavities and gum disease. A diagnosis of Sjögren's is extremely difficult: it has been known to take as long as two or even eight years!

Meanwhile, treatment is necessarily symptomatic. A special low-concentration eyewash containing cyclosporine, a powerful immuno-suppressant, may be prescribed, or an oral antimalarial like hydroxychloroquine. For dry mouth there are prescription drugs that stimulate the production of saliva: pilocarpine (Salagen); and regular dental check-ups are vital. There are also mechanical topical treatments: for the eyes, drops called 'artificial tears' (usually satisfactory) and for the mouth, 'artificial saliva' sprays (usually not satisfactory). It is possible to block the tear ducts surgically to retain moisture, and of course sufferers need to avoid smoke, strong winds and any form of airborne irritant, and to use eye make-up extremely sparingly. Sufferers should beware of proprietary over-the-counter products that promise to cure sore, reddened eyes. These contain *vasoconstrictors* that will make blood vessels constrict, aggravating the dryness and discomfort of Sjögren's.

Fibromyalgia

Fibromyalgia, or fibromyalgia syndrome (FMS), was only recognized by the American College of Rheumatology (ACR) and included in the official diagnostic manuals in 1990. The name derives from three Greek syllables: *fibro-* (fibrous or connective tissue), *my-* (muscle), *algos* (pain), but its most prominent symptom is debilitating fatigue. Some experts believe it is the same condition known as chronic fatigue syndrome, now usually called myalgic encephalitis or ME (more Greek, meaning 'brain inflammation').

Characteristically, the pain of FMS is spread throughout the body, not confined to joints. In addition people with FMS may experience disturbed sleep patterns, difficulty in concentrating, migraine headaches, anxiety and depression, hearing and seeing problems and heart-valve abnormalities (see box, 'Hole in the heart link to headaches' below). Things are usually worse in the morning. Some studies suggest that sufferers may also have unusual variations in hormonal or other biochemical patterns, and some also suffer from Raynaud's phenomenon. Brain-imaging technology confirms that FMS sufferers actually process pain signals differently from most people: their pain is amplified – like turning up the volume.

Hole in the heart link to headaches

Thousands of migraine sufferers (and this includes many of those diagnosed with FMS or ME) may have a small hole in the heart which can be corrected by a simple patch. A clinical trial currently in progress is investigating those who suffer from severe migraine accompanied by pins-and-needles and by a visual disturbance known as *aura* – flashing lights, bright spots, blind spots or like seeing through a snow storm. As many as a sixth of the 6 million UK migraine sufferers may fall into this category. Researchers believe that these migraine sufferers may have a common heart defect called patent formen ovale (PFO), shared with up to a quarter of the population, the majority totally unaware. A PFO is a hole, usually harmless, up to a centimetre across, between the two upper chambers of the heart. The researchers believe that in these cases some blood, which should be filtered through the lungs, may be bypassing them through the PFO, allowing chemicals that contribute to migraine to get to the brain.

The connection between holes in the heart and headaches was discovered serendipitously when a number of migraine sufferers who were among deep-sea divers with 'the bends' and stroke victims, underwent the patch procedure to correct their PFOs and discovered that their headaches had also disappeared.

Like the other disorders in this chapter, FMS can exist alone or with one or more CTDs. Up to a third of those with a CTD, including lupus, may have it. As with nearly all these conditions, the cause is unknown. There is some evidence of familial, probably genetic predisposition, with the likely trigger being a virus or other infection. Treatment is again targeted on symptoms. Unlike lupus, FMS does not respond to steroids, antimalarials or immunosuppressants, and NSAIDs are usually inadequate in the face of the severe pain, which may demand stronger painkilling drugs called *opiates*. Sometimes antidepressants seem to relieve the pain: either an older tricyclic drug called amitriptyline (Elavil) or one of the newer selective serotonin re-uptake inhibitors, or SSRIs (Prozac). These are usually given in lower doses than are required for anxiety or depression. Trials are going on to see if an anti-seizure drug, gabapentin (Neurontin), successful in reducing various sorts of nerve pain, might be effective.

To date the most successful ways of treating FMS are DIY. Sufferers learn to avoid extremes of cold or heat; physical or mental stress and either too much or, contrariwise, too little, exercise. A climate with warm, dry weather; regular, gentle cycling on the flat, or swimming in a heated pool is ideal. A physiotherapist may be able to devise a routine for FMS sufferers confined to British shores. Professional massage and acupuncture have helped some people.

Libman-Sacks endocarditis

Two more American physicians bequeathed their names to posterity in 1923 by describing a condition that is estimated to affect from 10 to 20 per cent of people with lupus.

In Chapter 1 we explained that the sheaths that line the heart and lungs are made of connective tissue and therefore vulnerable in lupus and other CTDs. Pericarditis – inflammation of the lining of the heart – is relatively common in lupus. *Endocarditis* involves the interior of the heart (*endo* is Greek for inside); in particular, the valves between chambers that regulate the flow of blood and prevent it going the wrong way. In Libman-Sacks endocarditis (LSE), tiny wart-like growths develop on the valves causing them to leak. Most people who develop it also have antiphospholipid antibodies (APS, or Hughes' syndrome, introduced in Chapter 5 and dealt with in detail in Chapter 10).

Doctors detect the possibility of LSE from listening to the heart (see box 'Listening to the heart' below). Heart valves affected by LSE cause a distinctive type of murmur behind the sound of the heartbeat. If the doctor thinks he or she can hear it he or she will probably confirm suspicions by asking the hospital to do an *echocardiograph*. Echocardiography passes sound waves into the chest, where they are reflected back to the instrument from the solid structures inside – an 'echo' of the structure. So the instrument forms a picture of the heart structure from the reflected sound waves (it is the same principle as radar or bats' sonar).

Listening to the heart

What does a family doctor, or indeed a specialist cardiologist hear when he or she sticks the stethoscope on your chest?

The heart is a synchronized pump – or, if you prefer it, a pair of pumps, synchronized to pass blood between their chambers and push it through the lungs and round the body. The skilled listener hears the one-way valves opening and shutting and blood being driven from one chamber in the heart to another. There are four distinct sounds in a normal heartbeat, usually described as making a noise rather like 'lop-dop'. The explosive consonants in 'lop-dop' are made by the valves opening and closing. A doctor learns to detect the sound of a healthy heart even though there may be slight variations in the patterns of sound. The doctor will note the speed of the beat. Does the heart race, or gallop even? He or she may also hear noises in between the distinct beats of the heart. These are called murmurs, and may indicate that the various valves are not working properly – for example, if they are leaking, and allowing some blood to go the wrong way.

These days there are many sophisticated ways of assessing the heart's performance: by plotting electrical impulses from the heart muscle – an *electrocardiogram*; by constructing images of the blood-flow – *magnetic resonance imaging (MRI)*; or by analysing the sounds – by echocardiograph. The stethoscope applied to the medically trained ear dominates front-line diagnosis because it is portable and doesn't need to be plugged in.

In itself LSE is not dangerous. Problems arise if the warts growing on the valves become infected. Various things can cause this but the most common is dental treatment. The mouth is a veritable hotbed of bacteria. And bacteria may get into the bloodstream if the body's internal mucous lining is broken in dentistry or in medical procedures like having a cervical smear or a *colonoscopy* – an internal investigation of the colon using a fibre-optic camera.

If an infection does occur in the heart valves the symptoms are fever, irregular heartbeat, difficulty in breathing and, if not treated, heart failure. To avoid this risk, LSE sufferers are prescribed antibiotics as a precautionary measure in advance of any risky dental or medical procedure.

Avascular necrosis

Avascular necrosis is the exception to the general rule that lupus, unlike rheumatoid arthritis, is not progressive, and does not do permanent damage to joints. (see box 'Cell death and recycling' below).

Cell death and recycling

For animals death is the end. If it comes during sleep, in the fullness of years, it is reckoned slightly better than if the animal is cut off in its prime, but it is still the end. It is a little different with cells. Cells are what living organisms are composed of – could be a tree, a goldfish or your old Uncle Harry – and they come and go in a constant cycle throughout the lifetime of that organism. It's as though Uncle Harry were a waterfall. (Don't be difficult; just try and imagine it.) The water in the waterfall is always changing, but the waterfall itself is still the same waterfall. That's how it is with the cells of the body. They are continuously produced (give or take a few exceptions like the corneal surface of the eye and some brain cells), go about their business and then pop off in an orderly and pre-programmed manner and are re-absorbed into the body – a sort of cell recycling. This end is known in medicine as apoptosis. You have met it in connection with the cells of the immune system, some of which fail to do this in autoimmune diseases.

Necrosis is another Greek word for death. (You will recognize this root in words like necropolis – a place where the dead are buried – or necrophilia – love attachment to a not very responsive person.) Necrosis is used in medicine to describe unscheduled and unhealthy death of cells or some part of the body: cell death as decay.

Joint pain is a feature of lupus for many. A small number also suffer actual damage to some part of the joint. The condition is known by a number of different names, most of which describe what it is *not*. It is not damage caused by trauma (atraumatic); it is not damage caused by infection (aseptic); what it is caused by is reduced blood supply, hence the name *avascular* necrosis. (Diminished blood supply leads to shortage of red blood cells, hence disruption to the delivery of their oxygen payload, and hence tissue damage.) There is uncertainty about how many lupus sufferers experience joint necrosis: it may be as many as 40 per cent, or it may be as few as 5.

Two parts of the joint may be damaged by avascular necrosis. First, bone – particularly the head of bone on load-bearing joints like the hips, knees and shoulders. (These are frequently the sites of other forms of arthritis: wear-and-tear osteoarthritis and rheumatoid arthritis.) When bone is affected the condition may be called *osteonecrosis*, adding the Greek term for bone to necrosis. Second, many more lupus patients suffer damage to tendons – the hawser-like structures that tether muscles to bone – caused by disrupted blood supply. This is known as tendon rupture, but is also described as 'fraying' or 'tearing'. The affected tendon does not need to be load-bearing and the most common site is the fingers. The rupture causes a sudden collapse of the bone supported by the tendon and can be quite alarming. If it is one of the bones of the hands the person may drop something; if a leg tendon, he or she may fall down. One patient described it: 'I've severed tendons like they were spaghetti, including the tendons in both of my thumbs – one of them twice. The latest was a *patellar tendon* in my knee. It happens when I am doing quite simple things; with one of my thumbs I was just picking up a bag of oranges! I've had more surgery than anybody I know.'

Lupus patients with a history of arthritis, blood disorders like anaemia, circulatory problems, high blood pressure, elevated choles-terol, diabetes, heavy drinking or (perish the thought) *smoking*, are more at risk of avascular necrosis. If bone is affected – osteonecrosis – the first symptom is likely to be pain in the joint itself, or possibly pain referred to a nearby area. If the necrosis is not checked there may also be pain at rest. Without treatment the necrosis causes actual loss of tissue in the joint, leading to collapse and fracture. To begin with the damage does not show up on X-rays, though it does on more sensitive imaging technologies.

Hopefully early intervention will prevent necrosis progressing to this point. The first-line treatment, once the problem is detected, is with drugs. In fact patients identified as being high-risk are usually offered prophylactic treatment to head off even the possibility of joint damage. Some risk factors can be reduced by modifying the lifestyle (cutting out cigarettes, alcohol and fatty junk foods), and others, like high blood pressure, anaemia and elevated cholesterol can be treated with relatively side-effect-free drugs. If bone damage is detected early a surgical procedure called *core decompression* will be recommended. A small core of tissue is withdrawn from inside the blood-deprived area of bone under anaesthetic to relieve the pressure, and also to encourage the formation of new, fine blood vessels and healthy bone. This procedure has been in use for more than thirty years and has a good record of avoiding more radical surgical treatment.

Once osteonecrosis reaches the stage at which it shows up on X-ray images, core decompression may be too late. Replacing the affected joint may then be necessary, especially in the case of a load-bearing joint like the hip or knee. This may sound radical but it has become an almost routine procedure for many people with osteoarthritis – the common wear-and-tear kind – and artificial knee and hip replacements have a very satisfactory history of restored movement and reduced pain. Ruptured tendons also have to be repaired by surgery.

Drug-induced lupus (DIL)

This last lupus-like condition is not so much lamb dressed up as wolf as a completely human-made wolf. To be precise, this is an *iatrogenic* form of lupus; meaning, caused by doctors, or medical treatment – *iatros* is Greek for physician – or, as one doctor puts it, 'Iatrogenic basically means "it's our fault".'

Mitch's story
Like a number of men who had worked hard, lived well and not taken enough exercise, Mitch's blood pressure crept up in middle age. Raised blood pressure increases the chances of heart disease and stroke and a good doctor always insists on correcting it. In Mitch's case modifying the lifestyle – cutting out salt, soft-pedalling the juice and getting out onto the golf course more –

didn't achieve adequate results. What's more, at one or his regular check-ups, his GP discovered he had an irregular heartbeat – one of the early signs of heart disease. She prescribed a drug to bring down the blood pressure and another to stabilize the heartbeat. At first, things improved and so did Mitch's handicap.

Some months later Mitch began to suffer from extreme fatigue. He told the cardiologist whom he was seeing and was told to take more exercise. 'How can I take more exercise when I feel dead beat from the moment I wake up', he complained to his wife. And then one morning he fell over at the first tee. His leg just gave way beneath him. He got up and tried to go on, but a few yards further down the fairway his other leg gave way. He went to his GP. She did a thorough examination and discovered that he was suffering from muscle weakness in both legs. His muscles were wasting away. She took blood and told Mitch she thought he had developed DIL. She stopped the drugs he had been taking and prescribed known, safe alternatives. She also sent Mitch off to a physiotherapist for a course of exercise to build up his wasted muscles.

More than one hundred different drugs have been reported as causing lupus-like conditions (see box 'Some drugs that induce lupus symptoms' opposite). The phenomenon was first noted in the 1940s. We know that some drugs (antibiotics, for example) can cause a flare in someone who already has lupus, but these drugs cause it in otherwise lupus-free people. The two drugs Mitch reacted to are those most often implicated, though they are not prescribed frequently these days.

What's the difference between drug-induced lupus (DIL) and the genuine article? Symptoms are usually, though not invariably, less severe: there may be fatigue, arthritis, widespread rashes, swollen lymph glands, pleurisy or pericarditis, but it is rare for the condition to cause kidney damage. Blood tests do not reveal the characteristic pattern of antibodies, but reveal some similarities and some differences, rather depending on the drug culprit causing the trouble. The principle difference is that all symptoms disappear soon after the drugs are withdrawn, leaving no lasting damage.

In the USA as many as 50,000 people are thought to suffer from DIL, though Graham Hughes says that, in his experience, it is 'rare' in the UK. Clearly the incidence of any iatrogenic condition is not a natural phenomenon. If the at-risk people and culprit drugs can be positively identified there should ideally be zero cases to report. However, it is not absolutely clear why some people develop DIL with certain drugs. There is a theory that some people metabolize drugs more slowly and may therefore be more vulnerable. It seems likely, as with lupus itself, that some genetic factor contributes to lupus being triggered by drugs.

Some drugs that induce lupus symptoms

- Hydralazine (blood pressure lowering agent)
- Procainamide, quinidine bisulphate (for irregular heart rhythm)
- Sulphasalazine (anti-inflammatory used for colitis and rheumatoid arthritis)
- Minocycline (antibiotic used for acne)
- Penicillamine (antibiotic)
- Isoniazid (antibiotic used for tuberculosis)
- Chlorpromazine (used for serious mental illness and severe nausea)
- Methyldopa (used for Parkinson's disease)
- Phenytoin (an anti-convulsant, used for epilepsy)

Some of the very latest drugs, for example biological agents developed to treat rheumatoid arthritis, have also been implicated in drug-induced lupus.

10

Lupus and pregnancy – the wolf and the ewe

Queen Anne's story

Queen Anne died in 1714, tormented as much by her physicians' misguided efforts at treatment as by her own agonizing illness. Her short life had been plagued by ill health; not least by an exhausting succession of miscarriages. In the first eighteen years of her marriage she had seventeen pregnancies, including eleven miscarriages (all the last nine), and only one child survived infancy. Since one of her primary aims in life, as the last of the Stuart line, a dynasty plagued by religious strife for nearly a hundred years, was to produce a Protestant heir, this was a bitter failure.

In his book *The Sickly Stuarts*, Professor Fredrick Holmes of the University of Kansas Medical Center in the USA, writes:

> Systemic lupus erythematosus remains the best explanation for Anne's ill-starred obstetric history and the disabling rheumatic disease she suffered in the last decade or so of her life . . . which led to her premature death from a cerebrovascular event – a stroke – common among sufferers of this disease.

In the view of Professor Holmes and Graham Hughes, Anne had lupus with antiphospholipid antibody syndrome (APS), a blood condition that, unchecked, causes pregnancies to fail between three and five months because of thrombosis: blood clots blocking the small blood vessels to the placenta which feeds the foetus. In modern times, if the antibody is identified a single aspirin a day can prevent miscarriage. Reflecting on this remedy Professor Holmes writes:

> In all likelihood in the early eighteenth century the equivalent was actually available as salicylic acid in herbal preparations containing willow bark, although its efficacy in Anne's condition could not have been known at the time . . . clearly Anne had the antiphospholipid antibody.

If Queen Anne's doctors had known what we know today history might have followed a different course; the house of Hanover might

84

not have inherited the throne of England and George III might not have lost the American colonies!

As recently as twenty-five years ago, doctors usually advised women with lupus not to get pregnant because recurrent miscarriage was a known symptom of the disease. But with a better understanding of the reasons behind these miscarriages the picture has changed. Studies of lupus pregnancies reveal that, whereas forty years ago less than half of them resulted in live births, these days between two-thirds and three-quarters are successful. And these figures are averages; in some centres, what is known as the 'take-home-baby' rate is even higher, although in about a quarter of lupus pregnancies there remains a risk of premature birth.

Facing up to the risks

Among the barrage of laboratory tests lupus patients undergo during diagnosis is one that is central to the outcome of pregnancy: the test for APS. We discussed this in Chapter 5. APS is now recognized as a distinct autoimmune disease in its own right, but whereas only about 5 per cent of the general population exhibit it, a very high percentage of lupus sufferers do. It is associated with increased risk of the formation of obstructive blood clots which in turn increase the danger of heart attack or stroke and, when they obstruct the blood supply to the placenta which nourishes the foetus, starve it of oxygen and cause miscarriage. The syndrome was first identified by Graham Hughes of St Thomas' Hospital and is also known as Hughes' Syndrome after him. (See Graham Hughes' book on lupus in 'Further reading'.)

People with APS also often have a wide range of other symptoms: seizures, migraine, joint pain and inflammation, avascular necrosis (see Chapter 9), leg ulcers, anaemia; most of them traceable to problems with circulation and thrombosis. All APS-related difficulties are made worse by smoking, high blood pressure, diabetes and high levels of cholesterol and other *lipids* (soluble fats) in the bloodstream.

Two further antibodies can cause trouble in pregnancy. One is called *anticardiolipin* (ACL), the other lupus anticoagulant (LAC). These two work in different ways to increase problems with the circulation and heart function, and the risk of miscarriage.

A diagnosis of APS requires both clinical symptoms – thrombosis or a history of miscarriage – and positive laboratory tests for ACL or LAC. As with other autoimmune diseases, the cause of APS is unknown, though studies support the idea of a genetic susceptibility triggered by a viral infection.

Any woman undertaking a pregnancy and diagnosed with APS, including those who also have lupus, will be put on an aggressive regime to correct the condition: drugs to lower high blood pressure, high cholesterol and other blood lipids and to control diabetes. The risk of blood clots can be reduced by aspirin or more powerful 'blood-thinning' drugs such as heparin.

It goes without saying that she will also be adjured to follow rigid pregnancy health behaviour *in spades*. She shouldn't smoke or drink, dabble with 'recreational' drugs, or any pharmacy product or supplement not prescribed by her doctor. She should pay particular attention to eating a balanced diet, follow her prescribed lupus medication to the letter and, above all, cling like a limpet to her rheumatology specialist as well as her obstetrician. Keeping lupus and APS under control during the pregnancy is absolutely central.

The medical team will inevitably rule out a home delivery. Women with lupus – or women with any chronic condition that poses a risk to either mother or child – need to be in a good hospital under specialist care when they give birth. There is an ever-present risk of premature birth with a lupus pregnancy and that means access to a unit equipped to care for the premature, or otherwise distressed, newborn.

Lupus drugs during pregnancy

It goes against instinct to be taking powerful drugs during pregnancy. And there are some drugs taken for lupus which are indeed counter-indicated, but surprisingly few. Steroids, probably prednisolone, even in quite large doses, do not appear to do harm. The mother's body breaks down this drug in the placenta in such a way that limits the amount reaching the foetus, though it is important that it doesn't lead to the mother gaining excessive weight. Some steroids do cross the placental barrier and may be used deliberately when an effect on the baby is intended. If a premature birth looks likely, a steroid called dextramethasone may be given to accelerate the development of the baby's lungs and reduce the breathing problems babies suffer when born early.

In the past antimalarials have been withdrawn during pregnancy because they also cross the placental barrier, but a recent French study suggests that possibly hydroxychloroquine may after all be safe, although a full examination of the eyes of the babies born in the study (vision is at risk from antimalarials) has not yet been completed. Powerful immunosuppressants are also usually avoided, although Graham Hughes reports that as many as 1,500 UK lupus patients had achieved successful pregnancies while on azathioprine. It is probably safer to say that the jury is still out on both drugs.

The immunosuppressant cyclophosphamide is definitely off limits, as are the high blood-pressure drugs known as *ACE inhibitors*, which can harm the baby if taken in the last six months (other blood-pressure drugs can be substituted) and the anti coagulant (blood-thinning) drug warfarin, which can harm the embryo in early pregnancy. (Heparin is the preferred alternative.)

Of course pregnancy and childbirth involve massive changes to hormone levels in a woman's body. It would be surprising were it not to have some effect upon a condition like lupus, which is known to be highly sensitive to the balance between various hormones. Even the most scrupulous care in monitoring the mother's health during pregnancy may not avoid a slight increase in the number of flares she experiences, but in general these are mild and easily controlled. There's a greater chance of a flare immediately after delivery when there is a sudden drop in progesterone – the hormone that has helped to maintain the pregnancy. To counter this, some doctors increase the dosage of steroids around the start of labour, gradually tapering it off only weeks after the birth. Others prefer to increase steroids only if and when a flare occurs. This is because at the time of birth it's important to consider what drugs may get into the mother's milk and so affect the baby. Breastfeeding has such wide-ranging benefits for the baby that the obstetric team does everything to make it easy for a new mother. And this may mean reducing drugs like antimalarials or aspirin that have helped keep the pregnancy flare-free shortly before the baby arrives. Once again, steroids do not pose a problem.

Risks to the baby

The biggest risk to a lupus birth is that it may occur too soon. As we have said, even with advanced modern treatment about a quarter of lupus births are premature. These days premature baby units are so sophisticated that we have become almost blasé about the problem, but it is still the goal of all good obstetricians that mothers go to full term: that is, between 35 and 37 weeks, or at very least until the baby weighs 1.5 kilos. Premature babies have difficulty in controlling their body temperature (and therefore have to spend a period in an incubator); they are also likely to have problems with breathing because their lungs are not fully developed, or to have difficulty in sucking. At the very least prematurity risks interfering with the bonding between mother and child that goes with established breastfeeding.

A number of risk factors common to all pregnancies can be more problematic for a lupus mother. One is a condition known as *pre-eclampsia* or toxaemia of pregnancy, when the kidneys, overwhelmed by the extra work of filtering the blood supply for an extra person, fail to eliminate all the waste products they usually clear from the bloodstream. Pre-eclampsia occurs late in pregnancy and is signalled by a rise in blood pressure, the presence of protein in the urine (normally filtered out by the kidneys) and oedema – fluid retention, causing puffy ankles, fingers and knees; another sign again that the kidneys are not coping.

As you might deduce, *pre*-eclampsia is the prelude to a condition called eclampsia, fortunately extremely rare these days because the warning signs are usually detected, when the inability of the kidneys to clear fluid from the tissues leads to seizures, unconsciousness and even death. Regular blood-pressure and urine checks usually pick up the danger signals in time, and since the delivery date is usually not far away, the doctors usually decide to induce the birth or even to perform a Caesarean section because, unchecked, the condition threatens the lives of both mother and child. Pre-eclampsia is a complication that affects between 5 and 7 per cent of all pregnancies but about 20 per cent of lupus pregnancies.

One other risk factor affects lupus pregnancies more than others. At about the fourteenth week of pregnancy the antenatal clinic usually tests the mother's blood for *alpha-foetoprotein (AFP)*. This is made almost exclusively by the baby's liver, and it is quite normal for levels to go up to some degree. However, exceptionally high concentrations seem to be associated with serious abnormalities of the baby's brain and spinal cord called *neural-tube defects (NTD)*. Only a minority of babies born following elevated AFP go on to develop NTD, but it is important that lupus mothers are monitored because they are more likely to develop high concentrations. The good news is that this doesn't seem to reflect a higher than normal chance of their babies having NTD; rather it seems related to the increased risk of those babies arriving prematurely. It also seems to go with higher doses of prednisolone – possibly for women with less well-controlled lupus.

Will the baby be all right?

You can see that in getting pregnant a woman with lupus is undertaking something that, while not as hazardous as it was forty years ago, is nevertheless not risk-free. The question all parents ask, including those without lupus, is: will nine months of caution and careful monitoring have their hoped-for reward? Will we have a healthy baby at the end of this pregnancy?

Lupus, as we have explained, is not directly inherited from mother to child. What does sometimes happen is that babies born to lupus mothers develop a short-lived lupus-related condition called *neonatal* lupus. Up to the moment of birth mother and baby have exchanged blood through the placenta, and what seems to happen is that some lupus antibodies have snuck across the placenta and got stranded in the baby where they inflame the baby's skin. Almost invariably the culprits are anti-Ro antibodies (a subset of ANA antibodies). Between 30 and 40 per cent of lupus patients have anti-Ro antibodies and between 10 and 20 per cent of those with the antibodies give birth to babies who exhibit neonatal lupus; at most 8 per cent of all lupus mothers. But it gives the new mother quite a turn because the baby develops a butterfly rash.

It must be emphasized that this is rare. Graham Hughes, who has seen thousands of lupus mothers through pregnancy, says he has only seen about a dozen in all his professional life. And it isn't real lupus. It's just a dying echo of the mother's lupus, and quickly clears up as the mother's antibodies disappear from the baby's blood.

Occasionally (in less than half the cases of neonatal lupus) the baby is born with a slight heart abnormality called *heart-block*; the electrical impulses of the heart are irregular making it sound as though it is stopping. But it doesn't. In itself slight heart *arrhythmias* are not life-threatening. (In older people they can be a warning of

89

something that *might* be life-threatening.) In a very few cases – we are now getting down to vanishingly small percentages – the arrhythmia is serious enough to require a pacemaker.

For those who don't want to get pregnant

Dora's story
Dora had a bad pregnancy in the early 1990s. She had blood clots and inflammation in the veins of her legs (*thrombophlebitis*) and fragments of blood clots in her lungs (*pulmonary emboli*). Her doctors advised her not to get pregnant again so she started taking the contraceptive pill. Then she developed some weird, really painful, red lumps on her legs. Her GP was nonplussed and referred her to the rheumatology department of the local hospital, which carried out blood tests and told Dora that she had both lupus and APS. The lumps, they told her, were *erythema nodosum* (Greek for 'red lumps'); a form of *vasculitis*, not exclusive to lupus sufferers though more common among them, which occasionally appeared on other parts of the body. The rheumatologist took Dora off the pill and advised a Dutch cap (the diaphragm).

If a woman with lupus decides she would rather not get pregnant, what should she do? To all appearances, controlled lupus has no effect on fertility, although periods are sometimes interrupted during a lupus flare. If she wants to avoid or plan pregnancy she needs some form of contraception. The female hormone oestrogen is known to exacerbate lupus symptoms and for twenty years the usual advice has been for lupus sufferers not to use the birth-control pill, especially those who experience the migraine and clotting problems associated with APS. However, a survey of patients at St Thomas' Hospital found that the same proportion of female lupus patients were taking oral contraceptives as of non-lupus mothers, with no apparent increase of side effects. Then, at the end of 2004, the Safety of Estrogens in Systemic Lupus Erythematosus National Assessment (SELENA) study in the USA reported similar results. Dr Michelle Petrie of Johns Hopkins Hospital told the annual scientific meeting of the American College of Rheumatology (ACR), 'This is a clinical trial you can take home with you. It will change the way you practice.' Henceforth oral contraceptives should be regarded as acceptable for the two-thirds of lupus patients who were not at risk of thrombosis, the trial concluded. This is good news because women with lupus are at higher-than-average risk of osteoporosis as a consequence of taking steroids, and oestrogen is known to protect against this condition.

Lupus patients who also have APS are still advised not to use any form of hormonal contraception – injections, patches or implants – because they may aggravate circulatory problems, high blood pressure, vasculitis and thrombosis. Some doctors believe that progestogen-only contraceptives are acceptable, but in general Sheldon Blau's advice remains: 'Shun all forms of hormonal contraception.' Intrauterine devices (IUDs) are also unsuitable for lupus patients because they have a higher likelihood of suffering perforation, bleeding or pelvic infections with the device. It comes down to good old barrier contraceptives: the diaphragm and condoms. These, of course, however tiresome they may be regarded, have the added advantage of protecting against sexually transmitted infection.

11
'Foretell the future' –
will the wolf one day become extinct?

Hippocrates, ancient Greek physician and father of medicine, gave his pupils modest goals: to help, or at least to do no harm. His instruction comes not from the celebrated oath – still taken by many medical students today – but from another of his writings called the *Epidemics*. Translated in full it reads: 'Declare the past, diagnose the present, foretell the future; practise these acts. As to diseases, make a habit of two things – to help, or at least to do no harm.'

Modern physicians have more ambitious goals: in reverse order – to bring relief, to cure and (the Holy Grail) wherever possible to prevent illness. In some cases – childhood diseases and infections, diseases caused by dietary deficiency – they have had spectacular success. In the case of the many forms of arthritis their success has been confined to bringing relief, controlling symptoms and preventing the worst damage. Cure is still a long way off; prevention even further.

As for 'foretelling the future' . . . doctors' ability to predict medical outcomes has made rapid strides in modern times. Researchers believe that there is hope that their understanding of autoimmune diseases like rheumatoid arthritis will provide greater control over outcomes in the not too distant future. Understanding opens the door to more precise, effective treatment, and side-effect-free treatment is the penultimate stop before cure. Prevention depends ultimately on understanding not only *what* goes wrong, but *why*, which, in the terms of the current hypothesis about autoimmune diseases, means identifying the triggers that set off the abnormal autoimmune reaction, and the genes that make some people susceptible in the first place. The answers, when they come, will probably emerge little by little, because it is possible that there will turn out to be more than one trigger, and certainly more than one susceptible gene.

This chapter will look into the crystal ball and see what shapes are emerging from the mist, or more prosaically, what avenues researchers are following.

New drugs in the pipeline

Drugs in the pipeline are not difficult to find on the Internet. It takes years to develop a new drug, absorbing vast sums of money, and only the hope of a matching profit if a new blockbuster makes it to market. So every candidate's progress is watched keenly by financial analysts as well as the medical fraternity. However, for every drug that reaches the final straight – being tested in humans for its safety and effectiveness – nine out of ten stumble on one of the numerous fences along the course. Of those that reach the finishing line, break the tape and go on sale, some may yet be withdrawn following a drug test (the racing metaphor is holding up quite well), as rare side effects only emerge after a drug has been taken by tens of thousands of patients for a lengthy period. That is what happened with the new COX-2 inhibitor Vioxx, which looked so promising for arthritis patients when first launched, but turned out to damage the hearts of some patients and was subsequently withdrawn. So the problem for drug manufacturers, doctors, patients and authors alike is which drug in the pipeline will stay the course? And to be honest, it's in the lap of the gods.

Here are some of those in the race:

Bromocriptine

This drug acts to reduce the release of a hormone called prolactin. As its name implies, prolactin encourages milk-production following childbirth, but as with so many hormones, it is produced and active in both sexes. High prolactin levels, associated with tiny tumours in the pituitary gland where it is released, lead to infertility by preventing menstruation and ovulation in young women, and bromocriptine has been used to treat this for some years. (Novel uses for drugs in this position start at an advantage because their safety has already been demonstrated in large numbers of patients.) The fact that lupus is a disease that strikes predominantly women of childbearing years has focused researchers' interest on hormones. High prolactin levels seem to stimulate the production of autoreactive antibodies in lupus, hence the idea that bringing them down with bromocriptine might help. It works in laboratory mice. Work in humans suggests that it could turn out to be on a par with hydroxychloroquine as a lupus treatment.

Prasterone

We looked at the role of hormones when considering the possible causes of lupus in Chapter 3. You first met prolactin there, and a form of androgen called dehydroepiandrosterone or DHEA, which is a precursor of both the male hormone testosterone and the female hormones that regulate fertility in women: oestrodiol and progesterone. DHEA levels are often lower than average in lupus patients of both sexes, which prompted the development of a synthetic version of DHEA called prasterone (Prastera). This has had a chequered career as it has undergone clinical testing. Lab mice with a lupus-like condition did well on it. It has been tested in humans with the goal of achieving a number of clinical improvements as well as confirmatory laboratory tests. A study reported in September 2004 noted a significant improvement in a wide range of lupus symptoms, with the exception of improved bone density, in the group taking prasterone compared with those on corticosteroids. Side effects of the drug were mostly mild and on the plus side it lowered the level of soluble fats like cholesterol in the bloodstream. By the time this book is published, it is possible the US authorities will have given prasterone a licence. If they do, prasterone will be the first *new* drug approved for lupus for forty years.

WARNING American expert Sheldon Blau alerts lupus sufferers to over-the-counter, so-called dietary supplements which profess to contain DHEA. Variously and unscientifically described as 'superhormones' or 'miracle drugs', they claim to promote weight loss, improve memory, fight infection, prevent cancer or heart disease and generally to make you live for ever with the body of a 20-year-old. Be advised: they won't. Sheldon Blau speaks for medical experts everywhere when he reminds us that licensed drugs have to undergo lengthy testing for safety, purity and effectiveness before they are let loose on the public. 'Supplements' don't.

Monoclonal antibodies

We learned in Chapter 3 on the causes of lupus that much of the damage in lupus is caused by antibodies, or B-lymphocytes, reacting to the body's own tissues – chiefly fragments from the interior of broken-down cells in the bloodstream. Attention has therefore been focused upon reducing the proliferation of these antibodies. On the principle of 'set a thief to catch a thief' scientists have tried to design tailor-made antibodies that will seek out and destroy those elements of the immune system that promote inflammation without reducing the parts that perform a protective function. These have worked well in laboratory mice bred to exhibit lupus-like symptoms.

'Synthetic' antibodies are constructed by cloning a single anti-body-producing cell, and are called *monoclonal antibodies (MoAbs)*. Two MoAbs are being investigated for the treatment of lupus. One called rituximab was approved some years ago for the treatment of a form of cancer called non-Hodgkin's lymphoma in which B-lymphocytes multiply beyond control. The MoAb attacks a marker on the surface of B-lymphocytes, which grow up to produce the autoimmune antibodies, which cause inflammation that does all the harm in conditions like rheumatoid arthritis and lupus. So it seems logical to see whether it would be effective in these conditions. In September 2004 researchers at the University of Rochester Medical Center in the USA reported that a single injection of rituximab gave 11 lupus patients, out of a total of 17, relief from a range of symptoms for a year or more. The improvement coincided with a drop in the number of B cells circulating in the patients' bloodstream. This was a very small trial and not randomly controlled (see Chapter 6, 'Randomized clinical trials (RCT) – the therapeutic Gold Standard'), so judgement must be provisional.

Another monoclonal antibody currently being studied in patients with lupus or rheumatoid arthritis strikes even earlier in the antibody-producing process. Its target is a recently discovered protein that stimulates B-lymphocytes, which grow up to produce the autoimmune antibodies ... and so on. A MoAb known provisionally as LymphoStat-B latches onto this self-explanatory B-lymphocyte stimulator (BlyS for short) and inhibits the development of harmful antibody-producing B cells. So far the MoAb has been shown to be side effect free.

Selective immuno-modulators

Lupus is an autoimmune disease, but the autoimmune system plays a vital protective role in the body so that even if you could, you wouldn't want to suppress it entirely. The goal is to find a drug that will be selective: a rapier rather than a blunderbuss; a drug that will remove the autoimmune antibodies causing the trouble while leaving the good antibodies to carry on with the positive work, vanquishing infection. Such drugs modify, or modulate, the immune system, hence the name immuno-modulators. The target of one such drug, code-named 'LJP 394' – trade name, Riquent – targets an antibody to a particular kind of DNA known as double-stranded DNA (hence an anti-dsDNA antibody), that shows up in the blood of lupus patients, especially when they have bouts of nephritis. So far it appears that the catchily named LJP 394 does reduce the quantity of anti-dsDNA antibodies and may also reduce the risk of nephritis.

Experimental treatments for kidney damage

The most serious manifestation of lupus is kidney inflammation – nephritis. If it proves impossible to 'head it off at the pass' there may come a stage when the only solution is a kidney transplant, and donor organs are in very short supply. A number of treatments short of replacement are being investigated.

A healthy body has inbuilt mechanisms for repairing damaged organs. One of the substances that stimulates this process has been identified and goes under another of those catchy pharmaceutical code names – BMP7. This stands for 'bone *morphogenetic* (form-generating) protein number 7', and a synthetic version of this protein has in fact been used successfully to speed the process of recovery in broken bones. Natural BMP7 is found in the kidneys. Inflammation, such as occurs in severe lupus, produces scar tissue known as renal fibrosis, and researchers have discovered that BMP7 can reverse this process and stimulate the production of new, healthy tissue. So far it's only been done in laboratory mice.

Two non-drug treatments have been tried for severe or unresponsive lupus which, while not surgical, might be classified under the heading 'heroic'. One is the use of targeted radiation – which is successful in preventing the recurrence of some cancers. Something called *total lymphoid irradiation (TLI)* targets the lymph nodes and other tissues where the lymphocytes – including the cells that grow up into the B cells that produce the antibodies . . . and so on – congregate. TLI appears to suppress some of the antibodies over-produced in lupus. It has been used successfully for some years to treat a potentially fatal form of lymphoma (cancers of the lymphatic system). Less frequently it has been tried for rheumatoid arthritis and multiple sclerosis. Its long-term safety and efficacy have not been established and, like some drug treatments, it makes patients more susceptible to infection. It is uncertain whether it will ultimately prove useful in severe and refractory lupus, which is only infrequently life-threatening.

The other non-drug treatment is *plasmapheresis*. This is a mechanical procedure rather like kidney dialysis, when the blood is circulated outside the body and harmful elements filtered out before the blood is returned. Plasma is the fluid in which various sorts of blood cell swim around. Pheresis (from the Greek for 'removal') is the process of filtering out things circulating in the blood. In the case of autoimmune diseases it can be used to remove some of the inflammatory antibodies and antigen-antibody complexes in the blood of lupus patients. So far it has only been used experimentally for rheumatoid arthritis and although it removed harmful antibodies and improved some symptoms, the results are not long-lasting. It doesn't appear to provide any improvement in the kidney problems which are the most severe manifestations of lupus.

And now for something completely different

On several occasions we have commented that the human body is, by and large, if not infallibly, a self-healing organism. It's what the autoimmune system, among others, is all about. In recent years, scientists have asked whether the processes the body uses to grow and develop as well as to heal, could be adapted to treat diseases that have so far foxed them. This is a step beyond making a drug in the laboratory that mimics a substance that is naturally active in the body, like a steroid. This is using the body's own cells as a cure (see box 'Chameleon stem cells' overleaf).

Stem cells may come from a donor, like a transplanted kidney, but preferably they are harvested from the patient's own blood. After the harvest the patient's abnormal mature cells are destroyed by use of a powerful immunosuppressant. This is the tricky stage because at that moment the patient is extremely vulnerable to infection having no functional immune system. Needless to say the procedure is carried out with the patient in hospital in protective isolation. Once the abnormal cells are cleansed the stem cells are reintroduced. Hopefully they mature, thrive and produce new, normally functioning cells for the patient. This procedure is called *autologous* (self-sourced) *haematopoietic* (blood-making) stem-cell transplantation.

97

Chameleon stem cells

Most adult body cells are specialists: as mature cells they are either specialist blood cells, muscle cells, brain cells. They cannot swap round and do a different job once they are mature. But cells start life as simpler, non-specialists known as stem cells. The most versatile stem cells are those in the embryo: the very beginning of life. Basic, dividing embryonic stem cells have the capacity to develop into all the different specialist cells a mature human body requires. Some embryonic stem cells are still present in the umbilical cord and that is why the UK has set up a unit to bank cord-blood harvested during birth. But even mature specialist cells, which are continually replacing themselves, start as immature forms and, in this state, can be encouraged to diversify if cleverly handled. It means harvesting immature stem cells from the site where they are produced: in the case of blood – white and red cells or platelets – this is in the bone marrow. Although blood cells are produced in the bone marrow, they can be harvested from blood by giving the patient something that encourages them to proliferate so that they spill out into, and can be picked up from, the bloodstream. They are then frozen in plastic bags with preservative – rather like smoked salmon in the supermarket – until they are needed.

It has only been used experimentally in specially selected patients since 1997, and has been successful for some cases of another disease of the immune system – non-Hodgkin's lymphoma – and is under consideration for rheumatoid arthritis. Because it is so risky it is only offered to patients with severe, drug-resistant, organ-threatening disease. At this moment that applies to very few lupus patients. However, this is almost certainly a form of therapy that has a very promising future.

Fundamental research in progress

The research discussed in this chapter is mostly about potential treatments being investigated in the clinic. But guiding new treatments is fundamental research into the disease process that goes on in laboratories, behind the scenes. There are a number of studies looking at ways of reducing the number of autoimmune B cells produced in lupus, and similar diseases, and also at understanding in what way they are different from B cells in people without Lupus. Studies are also going on to identify the genes that make people susceptible to lupus and other autoimmune diseases.

Dr Madeleine Devey of the Arthritis Research Campaign (ARC) believes that understanding genetics will eventually lead to much better targeted treatment for lupus:

> Therapy has improved markedly in recent years and the death rate of this potentially fatal condition has fallen. In the UK, at Imperial College, London, they are making a big effort to understand the genetics of lupus in mice, with the strong likelihood that these genes with have exact counterparts in humans.

Meanwhile, in the USA, researchers at the University of Minnesota recently announced that they have identified the first gene variant to be associated with lupus. Although it is found in approximately 16 per cent of unaffected Caucasians, it is much more common – nearly 25 per cent – among these with lupus or insulin-dependent diabetes, another autoimmune condition. Timothy Behrens, the principal investigator, says, 'This is the first time we have identified a variant that predisposes to many different autoimmune diseases.' Behrens believes that dozens of genes may well turn out to be responsible for lupus and that discovering the combination of these genes will be important to developing better diagnosis and treatment of the disease.

Glossary

Allergic   showing an unhealthy response to something as a result of previous exposure

Alpha-foetoprotein (AFP)   protein produced in the foetus' liver, picked up in the mother's blood, which reveals information on foetal development

Anaemia   shortage of oxygen-carrying red cells in the blood

Androgens   a general term for male sex hormones; testosterone is the principal male sex hormone

Angiotensin converting enzyme (ACE) inhibitor   blood-pressure-lowering drug

Ankylosing spondylitis   form of arthritis that affects the vertebrae

Antibodies   disease-fighting cells produced in response to a specific antigen

Anticardiolipin   antibody associated with blood-clotting problems

Anticoagulant   drugs that reduce a tendency for the blood to clot

Antigen   something that prompts antibody reaction

Antinuclear antibodies (ANA)   antibodies that react to material from the cell nucleus often present in connective tissue diseases

Antioxidant   molecule able to counteract the damaging effects of free oxygen atoms (free radicals) on the body

Antiphospholipid antibody syndrome (APS)   also Hughes' syndrome; a condition causing clots inside blood vessels predisposing women to miscarriage

Apoptosis   programmed cell-death

Arrhythmia   uneven heartbeat; an early sign of cardiovascular disease

Arthritis   inflammation of joints accompanied by pain and swelling; many varieties

Aura   visual disturbance that sometimes precedes migraine or seizure: flashing lights, bright or blind spots, blurred vision

Autoimmune disease   condition in which cells of the immune system (antibodies) attack the body's own tissues

Autologous   originating with the self; harvesting the patient's own blood or stem cells

Autoreactive   antibodies that act against the body's own tissues

Avascular necrosis bone or tendon damage caused by reduced blood supply

Bisphosphonates anti-osteoporosis drugs

Calcium antagonist blood-pressure-lowering drug acting on blood-vessel walls

Casein one of the proteins in cheese

Chronic condition that comes and goes; opposite of acute

Clusters incidence of disease concentrated in one location

Cognitive behaviour therapy (CBT) changing how someone thinks and evaluates events

Colonoscopy internal investigation of the colon (large bowel) with fibre-optic camera

Comparator standard treatment or drug against which new drug is assessed

Complement collections of proteins that support antibody activity

Compliance following medical instructions; opposite of non-compliance

Concordant having a characteristic in common; matching

Connective tissue diseases (CTD) group of diseases (including lupus) that affect related tissues widely distributed throughout the body

Core decompression surgical treatment for bone necrosis designed to stimulate healthy cell growth

Corticosteroid, cortisone powerful anti-inflammatory drug modelled on a naturally occurring human hormone, cortisol

Cyclo-oxygenase (COX) enzyme that stimulates the production of prostaglandins; painkillers that inhibit COX-2 selectively cause fewer gastric side effects

Cytokines chemical messengers that communicate between cells

Dehydroepiandrosterone (DHEA) precursor to the sex hormones testosterone in men and oestrodiol and progesterone in women, often below normal in lupus patients

Deoxyribonucleic-acid (DNA) material in genes that transmits hereditary information

Differential diagnosis evaluating a number of diagnoses and selecting the most likely

Diuretic drug that increases fluid excretion and helps lower blood pressure

Echocardiograph graphic representation of the interior of heart using sound waves

E-coli common bacteria (name of a species *genus* usually printed in Latin and italic)

Electrocardiogram graph of the electric impulses that regulate the heart

Endocarditis inflammation of the lining of the heart

Endorphins chemicals produced in the brain that reduce pain and increase well-being

Epidemiology study of disease in populations

Erythema nodosum form of blood-vessel inflammation (vasculitis) characterized by painful, reddish nodules

Erythrocyte red blood cell

Erythrocyte sedimentation rate (ESR) speed at which red cells in solution sink to the bottom of a test tube; indicator of unspecified infection or inflammation

Fibromyalgia rheumatic syndrome characterized by generalized muscle pain and fatigue

Genome total information for a living system contained in DNA sequences

Haematologist specialist in blood disorders

Haematopoietic producing blood cells

Haemophilia inherited, sex-linked, potentially fatal bleeding disorder (women carry it, men suffer it) caused by absence of blood-clotting factors

Heart-block heartbeat irregularities due to misfiring of electrical signals in the heart

Herpesviruses group of common viruses (chicken-pox, cold-sores, shingles) that, once caught, often recur; suspected of involvement in autoimmune diseases

Iatrogenic caused by doctors or medical treatment

Immune complex 'clumps' of warring antibody/antigen that cause damage to surrounding tissue

Incidence number of new cases of a disease

Leukaemia cancer of blood-producing tissue leading to over-production of abnormal white-cell forms and a reduction of normal blood cells

Lipids soluble fats circulating in the blood; high levels are associated with stroke and heart attack; cholesterol is a lipid

Lymphocyte white cell active in the immune system

Macular retinopathy damage caused by pigment deposited in the retina, the part of the eye that forms and relays images to the brain

Magnetic resonance imaging (MRI) diagnostic technique using radio-frequency pulses to create three-dimensional images of body tissues

Major histocompatibility complex (MHC) genes that code for which tissue types the body recognizes as compatible and which are rejected as foreign

Malar rash so-called 'butterfly' rash, usually facial, characteristic of lupus

Metabolize/metabolism biological process by which energy is extracted from oxygen and nutrients and waste products eliminated

Monoclonal antibodies (MoAbs) synthetic antibodies targeted on a single antigen

Morphogenetic form-generating; stimulating growth of new tissue

Myalgic encephalitis (ME) see fibromyalgia

Necrosis tissue damage through erosion, decay or rupture

Neonatal immediately after birth

Nephritis inflammation of the kidneys

Nephrologist specialist in kidney disease

Neural-tube defect (NTD) damage to the foetal brain or spinal cord

Non-compliance see compliance

Oedema accumulation of fluid in tissues spaces

Oestrogen one of the hormones regulating the female menstrual cycle

Ophthalmologist specialist in eye disease

Opiates group of powerful painkillers (e.g. morphine)

Osteoarthritis joint pain and deformity caused by wear and tear

Osteonecrosis bone-cell decay or 'death'

Osteoporosis loss of bone density leading to brittle bone and easy fracture

Patellar tendon tendon tethering the quadriceps muscle at the front of the knee and maintaining the stability of the joint upon which the knee-cap (patella) is set

Pericarditis inflammation of the membrane surrounding the heart

Pericardium outer membrane surrounding the heart

Photosensitive abnormal or extreme reaction to light

Placebo dummy pill used in clinical trials to compare the effectiveness of an active drug

Placebo effect   improvement demonstrated by patients taking a dummy pill

Plasmapheresis   filtering blood outside the body to remove abnormal cells

Platelet   blood cell that initiates clotting; also thrombocyte (clotting cell)

Pleura   membrane surrounding the lungs

Pleurisy   inflammation of the membrane surrounding the lungs

Polymyositis, dermatomyositis (PM-DM)   form of CTD, often occurring together, characterized by generalized muscle and skin inflammation

Pre-eclampsia   failure of the kidneys to filter waste products from the body during the last phase of pregnancy

Prevalence   total number of those with a condition in a given population

Prognosis   predicted outcome of a disease or treatment

Prostaglandins; prostaglandin-inhibitors   substances that contribute to, and modify inflammation and blood-clotting; drugs like aspirin and NSAIDS that inhibit them

Psoralen   chemical found in some plants that increases photosensitivity

Pulmonary emboli   fragments of blood clots that obstruct the lungs

Pulse therapy   administering a drug in 'bursts' via intravenous injection

Randomized, controlled trials (RCT); randomized, placebo-controlled, double-blind trials   trials where patients are randomly assigned to either an active or a comparator (usually standard) treatment; trials where treatment is tested against a patient group taking a dummy pill, and neither patients nor administering physicians know which is which

Raynaud's phenomenon or syndrome   condition characterized by numb, blue fingers and toes, caused by vasospasm in response to cold or other stimuli

Rheumatoid arthritis   inflammatory CTD principally affecting multi-directional (synovial) joints, also blood vessels and membranes

Rheumatoid factor   antibody found in the blood of about 80 per cent of rheumatoid arthritis patients and some with other inflammatory conditions

Rheumatologist specialist in inflammatory conditions

Ribonucleic acid (RNA) building-block chemicals that transfer genetic information in viruses

Salmonella group of germs (bacilli) associated with food poisoning in humans

Sclerosis, scleroderma hardening of connective tissue or skin

Sicca syndrome dry eyes and mouth caused by blockage of fluid-secreting ducts by inflammation; see also Sjögren's syndrome

Sjögren's syndrome an autoimmune disease that reduces the secretions of many glands of the body, resulting in severe dryness of the eyes, mouth and vagina

Statin lipid-lowering drug that has other beneficial side effects

Systemic affecting organs throughout the body

Systemic lupus erythematosus (SLE) full name and acronym of lupus

Therapeutics science of treating illness with drugs

Thrombocyte cell that promotes clotting; see platelet

Thrombophlebitis inflammation of veins, often in legs

Tinnitus persistent ringing in the ears

T-lymphocytes (also B-lymphocytes) subclasses of lymphocytes with different functions in the immune process

Total lymphoid irradiation (TLI) irradiation of lymph nodes with aim of reducing abnormal lymphocytes that congregate there

Vasculitis inflammation of blood vessels

Vasoconstrictors drugs that cause blood vessels to constrict

Vasospasm spasmodic contraction, closing down of small blood vessels

Vesicles small bladder-like cavities

Useful addresses

Research and support organizations in the UK

There are patient-support organizations for lupus all over the world. National associations will usually put you in touch with local groups, or, if you search the Internet, you may be able to locate them directly. (The West Midlands of the UK is particularly well served.) In addition to patient-support, some organizations focus on research. Their scope may be broader than lupus and embrace other forms of inflammatory arthritis, connective tissue diseases or autoimmune diseases. We have included some of these like the Arthritis Research Campaign (ARC) if they produce information directed to the health consumer.

Arthritis Care
18 Stephenson Way
London NW1 2HD
Tel.: 020 7380 6500
Website: www.arthritiscare.org.uk
Arthritis Care produces a newsletter called *Arthritis News*. Details from their website, or phone 0845 600 6868. It also carries a list of support organizations in this country and worldwide.

The Arthritis Research Campaign (ARC)
Copeman House
St Mary's Court
St Mary's Gate
Chesterfield
Derbyshire S41 7TD
Tel.: 0870 850 5000
Website: www.arc.org.uk
ARC's website provides details of research centres and scientific information about all forms of arthritis. ARC also publishes leaflets and a magazine called *Arthritis Today*.

The College of Health
St Margaret's House
21 Old Ford Road
London E2 9PL
Tel.: 020 8983 1225
Website: www.collegeofhealth.org.uk
Represents the interests of NHS patients in the UK.

Hughes' Syndrome Foundation
The Rayne Institute
St Thomas' Hospital
London SE1 7EH
Tel.: 020 7188 8217
Website: www.hughes-syndrome.org

Lupus UK
St James House
Eastern Road
Romford
Essex RM1 3NH
Tel.: 01708 731251
Website: www.lupusuk.com
A comprehensive site with news, information, advice, support contacts and details of research in progress.

St Thomas' Lupus Trust
The Louise Coote Lupus Unit
Gassiot House
St Thomas' Hospital
London SE1 7EH
Tel.: 020 7188 3562

Some lupus organizations overseas

Australia

Lupus Australia Foundation
Level 2
247–251 Flinders Lane
Melbourne
VIC 3000
Australia

USEFUL ADDRESSES

Tel.: 03 9650 5348
Website www.lupusvic.org.au
A number of linked Australian state lupus-support organizations are
at this Melbourne address.

Canada

Lupus Canada
590 Alden Road
Suite 211
Markham
ON L3R 8NT
Tel.: 905 313 00004
Toll free: 1 800 661 1468
Email: www.lupuscanada.org
A number of linked Canadian provinces' lupus organizations are
listed on the website. The Lupus Society of Alberta website
(www.lupus.ab.ca) features a wonderful animated cartoon that
explains lupus antibody behaviour and makes you laugh!

Europe

European Lupus Erythematosus Federation (ELEF)
St James House
Eastern Road
Romford
Essex RM1 3NH
Tel.: (44) 1708 731271
Website: www.elef.rheumanet.org

USA

Arthritis Foundation
P.O. Box 7669
Atlanta, GA 30357-0669
Tel.: 404 872 7100
Website: www.arthritis.org
A massive website covering all forms of arthritis with information,
news stories, the latest research, patient histories and details of local
offices all over America.

Lupus Foundation of America
2000 L. Street, NW
Suite 710
Washington
DC 20036
Tel.: 202 349 1156
Website: www.lupus.org
An organization with many ramifications: patient support and chat rooms, news, information, advice and patient contact networks, clinical trials recruiting, reading list. The scope is endless.

Lupus and family on the Internet

There are a large number of active associations and major university departments in the USA which present themselves instantly with an Internet search. We list below some of those we found most helpful (and entertaining). Where we direct you to a particular page on a site we indicate what it is about rather than the parent site's name.

Advice on things that increase photosensitivity
www.emedicine.com/derm/topic108.htm

The American Autoimmune Related Diseases Association
www.aarda.org

History of the immune system
www.keratin.com/am/amindex.shtml

Lupus Alberta (Canada) animated cartoon on what happens in lupus: amuses and informs
www.lupus.ab.ca/viewpage.asp?p=RESOURCES-FLASH&n=1

National institute of Arthritis, Musculoskeletal and Skin Diseases
www.niams.nih.gov

Fraud, scams, alerts about unsubstantiated medical claims
www.quackwatch.org

Tips on Internet searching

The Internet is a source of such endless information that the only problem is sorting the wheat from the chaff. Some useful tips: the boxes at the side of the page are paid for, so may have an axe to grind. The suffix .org implies a charity or an organization whose primary focus is not commercial. The suffix .ac or .edu implies an academic or educational site, likely to be well informed but possibly narrow or esoteric in focus. Beware of jazzy, all-singing, all-dancing sites. They probably aren't serious. If you haven't yet found the impressive search engine Google, try it.

If you aren't on-line, go to the public library and browse for free. There is information, support and the experience of other people with lupus out there to share.

Further reading

* Author recommendation

* Sheldon Paul Blau and Dodo Schultz, *Living with Lupus: The Complete Guide*, Da Capo Press, 2nd rev. edn, 2004

Triona Holden, *Living with Hughes Syndrome: Your Essential Guide to 'Sticky Blood'*, Sheldon Press, 2002

Triona Holden and Graham Hughes, *Talking about Lupus: What to Do and How to Cope*, Piatkus Books, 2004

* Graham Hughes, *Lupus, the Facts*, Oxford University Press, 2000

Maureen Pratt, David Hallegua and Daniel J. Wallace, *Taking Charge of Lupus: How to Manage the Disease and Make the Most of Your Life*, New American Library, 2002

The following recommended US publications may be obtained directly from Lupus UK, St James House, Eastern Road, Romford, Essex RM1 3NH. Tel: 01708 731251 and on-line at www.lupusuk. com

Henrietta Aladjem (founder of the Lupus Foundation of America), *The Challenges of Lupus: Insights and Hope*, Avery, 1999

Robert G. Lahita, Robert H. Phillips, *Lupus: Everything You Need to Know*, Avery, 1998

Lupus: A GP Guide to Diagnosis, Lupus UK, 2000

Dr Robert H. Phillips, *Coping with Lupus*, Avery, 2001

Daniel J. Wallace, *The Lupus Book: A Guide for Patients and Their Families*, rev. edn, Oxford University Press, 2000

Butterfly Traveller, ELEF and Novartis Pharma Verlag, 2000
A medical phrase book for the lupus patient and other travellers, in 12 different languages.

Living with Lupus (video), Lupus UK
A guide for patients with SLE (systemic lupus erythematosus).

Index

relaxation 72
respiratory system 7–8, 34–5
rheumatoid arthritis xi, 3, 22,
33–4, 98; fats and 69; finger
flexor tendonitis 44;
mistaking symptoms for 6–7
Rogerius 14

Safety of Estrogens in
Systemic Lupus
Erythematosus National
Assessment 90
St Thomas' Hospital 42–3
Sennert 14
Sickly Stuarts, The (Holmes)
84
Sjögren's (Henrik) syndrome
44, 65, 74–5
smoking 29

social life 67
sores 32
stem-cell treatment 97–8
steroids *see* corticosteroids
sunlight: beliefs about xi–xii
support groups 67
swelling: from kidney problems
8; symptoms 4–5

tiredness xi; fibromyalgia 75–6;
management of 62–3; as
symptoms 1, 30
total lymphoid irradiation (TLI)
96
treatment *see* drug treatments

vision: antimalarial drugs 54–5;
aura 76